Statins - Emerging Trends in Heart and Cancer Treatment

Edited by Rakesh Sharma

Published in London, United Kingdom

Statins - Emerging Trends in Heart and Cancer Treatment
http://dx.doi.org/10.5772/intechopen.1007260
Edited by Rakesh Sharma

Contributors
Luis Miguel Guerrero Cepeda, María Augusta Tinoco Lara, Oluwafemi Ajoyemi Ala, Rakesh Sharma, Tatjana Ábel, Éva Csajbókné Csobod

First published in London, United Kingdom, 2026 by IntechOpen
IntechOpen is the global imprint of INTECHOPEN LIMITED, registered in England and Wales, registration number: 11086078, 167-169 Great Portland Street, London, W1W 5PF, United Kingdom

For EU product safety concerns: IN TECH d.o.o., Prolaz Marije Krucifikse Kozulić 3, 51000 Rijeka, Croatia, info@intechopen.com or visit our website at intechopen.com.

British Library Cataloguing-in-Publication Data
A catalogue record for this book is available from the British Library

Statins - Emerging Trends in Heart and Cancer Treatment
Edited by Rakesh Sharma
p. cm.
Print ISBN 978-1-83635-235-8
Online ISBN 978-1-83635-234-1
eBook (PDF) ISBN 978-1-83635-236-5

Meet the editor

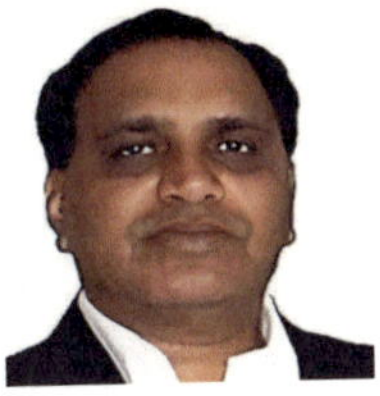

Professor Rakesh Sharma has an academic background in BAMS traditional medicine, a Master of Science in biochemistry and applied nutrition (NIN), a Ph.D. in medical biochemistry, and a second Ph.D. in biomedical engineering (MRI) at IIT/AIIMS Delhi. Dr. Rakesh Sharma conducted research at UCSF, Baylor College, Columbia University, the National High Field Magnetic Resonance (FSU), and Massachusetts General Hospital in Boston, focusing on medical imaging and nanotechnology. Dr. Rakesh Sharma taught biochemistry at medical colleges in India and biomedical engineering and MRI at FSU. Dr Rakesh Sharma has published over 170 research articles, 90 peer-reviewed conference papers, and 6 books.

Contents

Preface **IX**

Section 1
Statin Mechanisms and Sex-Differences **1**

Chapter 1 **3**
Perspective Chapter: Statins Use in Cancer Treatment – Unraveling the Mechanisms and Future Therapeutic Frontiers
by Oluwafemi Ajoyemi Ala

Chapter 2 **41**
Perspective Chapter: Sex Differences during Statin Therapy in Patients with Elevated Risk of Cardiovascular Disease and Cancer
by Tatjana Ábel and Éva Csajbókné Csobod

Section 2
Nanotechnology and Cardio-Oncology **63**

Chapter 3 **65**
Statin Nanoformulation Methods in Cancer Theranosis: Trimodal Therapy
by Rakesh Sharma

Chapter 4 **93**
Pleiotropic Effects of High-Potency Statins and their Impact on Cardio-Oncology
by María Augusta Tinoco Lara and Luis Miguel Guerrero Cepeda

Preface

This book, *Statins – Emerging Trends in Heart and Cancer Treatment,* presents the current status of statins as repurposed drugs to reduce cholesterol and cardiotoxicity caused in cancer patients. Various clinical trials and observations continue to place statins under scrutiny, prompting calls for extensive clinical studies.

Statins have been used for cardiovascular protection and lipid-lowering for the past half-century. However, over four to five years of continuous use of statins has been in controversy over statin adverse or toxic carcinogenic effects, which has often caught the attention of the public about its continuous daily use, while governmental agencies and authorities remained silent spectators with limited clinical evidence of statin safety. The success of optimal low-dose statin use over the years in lipid-lowering and myocardial oxygen-utilization effects has motivated pharmaceutical manufacturers to continuously push hard the statin drugs as monotherapy for improving heart health, cardiovascular blood circulation, and safe repurposed adjunct statins given with chemotherapy, radiotherapy, immunotherapy, and antioxidants in combination therapy to cancer survivors. On the other hand, some statins have been restricted to low doses of simvastatin, atorvastatin, and rosuvastatin to avoid muscle weakness.

The present book highlights the growing potential of existing and emerging statin drugs in both high cholesterol management and enhancing oxygen utilization in the cardiovascular system. Another major focus is statins as repurposed anticancer adjunct therapy.

The book is presented in two sections.

Section 1 focuses on an introduction to statins, lipid-lowering concepts, transformed prenylation mechanism of repurposed statin anticancer actions, such as antiproliferation, anti-inflammatory, anti-apoptosis, anti-autophagy, antioxidant, anti-immunogenic, and anti-cell cycle control mechanisms, to define the meaning of 'repurposed statins' apart from statin-induced cholesterol-lowering HMG-CoA reductase enzyme inhibition action.

The routine use of statins in patients at risk of diabetes mellitus (T2DM) or metabolic dysfunction-associated steatotic liver disease (MASLD) shows the differences in males and females for lipid-lowering and reduced oxygen among cancer survivors.

Section 2 focuses on synergistic effects, including anti-inflammatory, antioxidant, endothelial-protective, and antithrombotic properties. These effects enhance the benefits of different statins when combined with chemotherapies, immunotherapies, targeted therapies, and cell-cycle control-point therapies.

The emerging field of nanotechnology is highlighted in the development of statin-based nanoformulations for 'trimodal therapy'. Different pleiotropic factors influence the anti-inflammatory, antioxidant, endothelial-protective, and antithrombotic properties. The nanoformulations show benefits in cardiovascular prevention, along with lipid lowering, when combined with statins administered and beyond in statin-based combination cancer therapies given to cancer patients.

The *Perspective Chapter: Statins Use in Cancer Treatment – Unraveling the Mechanisms and Future Therapeutic Frontiers* compiles a global effort on defining different types of statins with their cardiovascular protection mechanisms in cancer survivors with specific focus on newly identified statin-repurposed mechanisms of synergistic characteristics as stimulators of apoptosis and autophagy with antiproliferative, anti-angiogenic, anti-immunogenic, anti-inflammatory, anti-cell growth and CAR-T therapeutic potentials in tumor cells to enhance the patient outcomes as tumor growth or recurrence predictors, monitors and biosensors. The chapter also focuses on unmet challenges, hype, the need for extensive research and clinical trials, and investigations to justify statins as potential options in cancer treatment.

Chapter 2, *Perspective Chapter: Sex Differences during Statin Therapy in Patients with Elevated Risk of Cardiovascular Disease and Cancer*, recommends the latest guidelines on statin therapy for male vs female patients with established cardiovascular disease (CVD), type 2 diabetes mellitus (T2DM), or metabolic dysfunction-associated steatotic liver disease (MASLD). The potential of statin actions is highlighted among males and females as possible sex differences in the effect of statin treatment on the development of different cancer types and CVD risk factors in patients with T2DM and MASLD.

Chapter 3, *Statin Nanoformulation Methods in Cancer Theranosis: Trimodal Therapy,* presents several preclinical evidences and clinical applications of statin use in oncology with emphasis on the low solubility and bioavailability of statins given with chemo-radiotherapy 'trimodal' drugs. The statin-chemodrug nanoformulations as nanomedicines enhance statin and chemodrug delivery, solubility, stability, and targeting, thereby achieving maximum anticancer therapeutic efficacy with maximum accumulation of nanomedicines in tumors, without any side effects. The author proposes and advocates "Trimodal Therapy" in the present chapter on the development of statin-loaded nanoformulations of liposomes, micelles, polymeric beads filled with chemo-radiotherapy drugs with immunotherapy and targeted therapy drugs as 'hybrid nanomedicines' or 'trimodal therapy'. The chapter also describes nanodelivery applications and anticancer properties in tumors to improve cancer treatment and better patient outcomes. The 'hybrid nano-drug' controlled delivery of statins with two or more anticancer drugs is state-of-the-art to enhance the anticancer effects and simultaneously reduce the cardiotoxicity, cytotoxicity, drug resistance, and tumor recurrence to enhance the overall clinical and patient outcomes.

Chapter 4, *Pleiotropic Effects of High-Potency Statins and their Impact on Cardio-Oncology*, reviews statins for their pleiotropic qualities beyond the benefit of lowering cholesterol. These statins protect the cardiovascular system by having anti-inflammatory, antioxidant, endothelial-protective, and antithrombotic properties. Statins have the potential to lessen chemotherapy-induced cardiotoxicity and androgen deprivation effects important in the field of cardio-oncology. Statins H maintain the left ventricular ejection fraction (LVEF) and lower the incidence of chemotherapy-associated cardiac dysfunction. Statins influence tumor growth, angiogenesis, and metastasis, exerting anticancer effects, and should be used more widely in oncology to assess their long-term effects on cardiovascular and cancer outcomes. The author emphasizes the necessity for individualized treatment plans in oncology.

The authors hope this book will meet the needs and interests of active researchers, scientists, pharmacologists, statin manufacturers, clinical practitioners, and academic physicians.

Rakesh Sharma
Government Medical College Saharanpur,
Saharanpur, India

Radhagovind Hospital,
Meerut, India

Section 1

Statin Mechanisms and Sex-Differences

Chapter 1

Perspective Chapter: Statins Use in Cancer Treatment – Unraveling the Mechanisms and Future Therapeutic Frontiers

Oluwafemi Ajoyemi Ala

Abstract

This chapter investigates the expanding role of statins as adjunctive agents in cancer therapy, offering a comprehensive synthesis of their molecular mechanisms, therapeutic relevance, and future clinical potential. Initially developed for lipid-lowering purposes, statins have demonstrated pleiotropic anti-cancer properties, exerting effects through modulation of critical oncogenic signaling pathways such as Ras, Rho, and NF-κB. These interactions contribute to the inhibition of tumor proliferation, suppression of angiogenesis, induction of apoptosis, and modulation of immune responses. Emphasis is placed on the organ-specific implications of statin therapy, with a detailed examination of their effects across a range of malignancies including breast, prostate, lung, colorectal, pancreatic, hepatic, and pulmonary cancers. The chapter integrates findings from preclinical models and clinical studies, highlighting the variability in therapeutic response across cancer types. Special focus is given to the synergistic potential of statins when combined with conventional chemotherapeutics, targeted therapies, and immunotherapies, particularly in overcoming resistance and enhancing treatment efficacy. Furthermore, the discussion addresses key challenges such as optimal dosing strategies, adverse effect management, and drug–drug interactions, advocating for precision oncology approaches that incorporate pharmacogenomic profiling and patient stratification. Emerging avenues such as nanoparticle-based drug delivery and personalized statin regimens are explored for their potential to maximize therapeutic outcomes while minimizing toxicity. Concluding with a call for rigorous, large-scale clinical trials, this chapter aims to provide a scientific basis for integrating statins into the evolving landscape of oncology, offering novel insights for researchers and clinicians pursuing innovative, evidence-based cancer treatment strategies.

Keywords: statins, cancer therapy, oncoproteins, angiogenesis, apoptosis, immune modulation, combination therapy, personalized medicine, drug repurposing, precision oncology

1. Introduction

1.1 Brief background of statins in medicine

Statins are a widely prescribed class of lipid-lowering agents with proven efficacy in managing dyslipidemia and reducing cardiovascular morbidity and mortality [1, 2]. As seen in **Figure 1**, their primary mechanism involves the competitive inhibition of the enzyme HMG-CoA reductase (3-hydroxy-3-methyl-glutaryl-coenzyme A reductase), a key regulatory catalyst in the hepatic mevalonate pathway responsible for endogenous cholesterol biosynthesis [3, 4]. By obstructing the conversion of HMG-CoA to mevalonate, statins effectively decrease intracellular cholesterol synthesis, triggering a compensatory up-regulation of low-density lipoprotein (LDL) receptors on hepatocytes [5].

Several statins have been developed for clinical use, including simvastatin, atorvastatin, and rosuvastatin, each differing in potency, bioavailability, and metabolic profile, as exemplified in their different structures as seen in **Figure 2** [6, 8].

1.2 Rationale for investigating statins in cancer treatment

Cancer is a multifactorial disease characterized by the uncontrolled proliferation and survival of abnormal cells, which can invade neighboring tissues and spread to distant organs through the lymphatic and circulatory systems. This progression is driven by genetic and epigenetic alterations that disrupt normal cellular regulation, leading to oncogene activation and tumor suppressor gene silencing. Statins, traditionally used for managing dyslipidemia and preventing cardiovascular diseases, have gained increasing attention in oncology due to their potential to modulate key aspects of cancer biology, offering a novel avenue for cancer prevention and treatment [9, 10].

Statins exert their primary effect by inhibiting HMG-CoA reductase, a key enzyme in the mevalonate pathway, which is essential for cholesterol biosynthesis. **Figure 3** explains that beyond the cholesterol-lowering actions of statins, statins induce a variety of pleiotropic effects, including the inhibition of cell proliferation and induction of apoptosis in cancer cells [11]. This is particularly relevant in hormone-sensitive malignancies, such as prostate cancer, where statins may enhance the efficacy of androgen deprivation therapy (ADT). By limiting the cholesterol

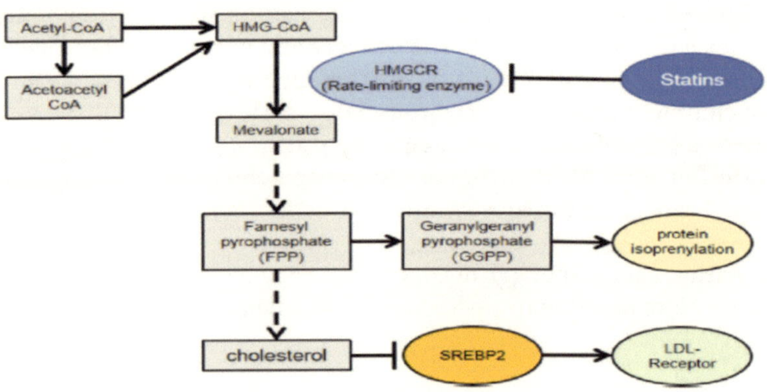

Figure 1.
Importance of statins in HMG CoA reductase blockade in mevalonate pathway [3, 4].

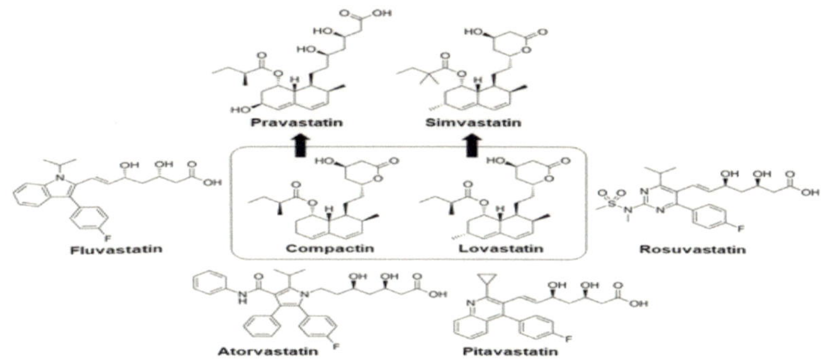

Figure 2.
Some structural examples of statins [6, 7].

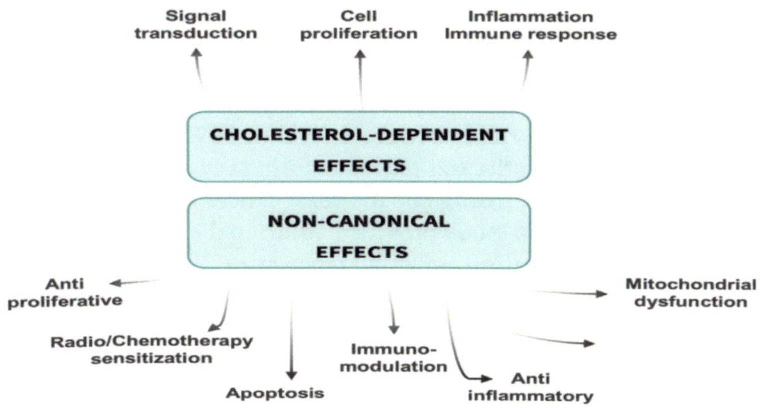

Figure 3.
Statins use in the field of clinical anti-tumor studies [11–13].

precursor pool required for steroid hormone biosynthesis, statins help prevent tumor adaptation under ADT, potentially improving therapeutic outcomes as seen in the **Figure 3** [11, 12].

By targeting endothelial function and the degradation of the extracellular matrix, statins exhibit potent anti-metastatic effects and a promising therapeutic adjunct that could prevent the spread of malignancies to other organs and optimize patient outcomes in cancer management [13].

1.3 Mechanisms of action in cancer cells

Statins exert their anticancer activity primarily through the inhibition of HMG-CoA reductase, a pivotal enzyme in the mevalonate pathway responsible not only for cholesterol biosynthesis but also for producing essential isoprenoid intermediates [14, 15]. While cholesterol is a precursor for steroid hormones, including androgens, the suppression of its synthesis by statins has drawn clinical interest for its potential to delay disease progression in hormone-sensitive malignancies, notably prostate cancer. Emerging clinical evidence suggests that lowering cholesterol levels can interfere with intra-tumoral androgen synthesis, thus enhancing the efficacy of androgen deprivation therapy (ADT) and potentially delaying the onset of castration resistance [16].

Beyond cholesterol regulation, the mevalonate pathway also generates isoprenoids such as farnesyl pyrophosphate and geranylgeranyl pyrophosphate, which are vital for the post-translational prenylation of small GTP-binding proteins like Ras, Rho, and Rac (Ras-related C3 botulinum toxin substrate). These proteins are key drivers of cell cycle progression, survival signaling, and metastatic behavior [17, 18]. By inhibiting isoprenoid synthesis, statins impede the activation and membrane localization of these oncogenic proteins, thereby curbing proliferative signaling and enhancing apoptotic sensitivity in cancer cells [17].

Although certain preclinical studies have identified statins, such as pitavastatin, as selectively cytotoxic to tumor cells—particularly those harboring PTEN (Phosphatase and Tensin Homolog) mutations—their true clinical potential lies in their ability to simultaneously disrupt proliferative signaling and steroidogenesis pathways without significantly harming normal tissues [18]. This multifaceted mechanism reinforces the rationale for incorporating statins into cancer therapy, especially in hormonally driven cancers where cholesterol and its derivatives fuel tumor progression.

Furthermore, statins have shown a strong association with improved outcomes in breast cancer, particularly in aggressive subtypes like triple-negative breast cancer (TNBC). A pivotal study published in Cancer reported that statin use improved breast cancer-specific survival by 58% and overall survival by 30% [19]. Furthermore, statins' cardioprotective properties mitigate chemotherapy-induced cardiac damage, enhancing their value as adjunctive agents in breast cancer therapy [20].

A Mendelian randomization study provided additional evidence for statins' role in reducing cancer cell proliferation and recurrence rates. These findings underscore the potential of statins as modulators of tumor progression and recurrence in breast cancer patients [21].

2. Mechanisms of statins in cancer therapy

Statins can have anti-cancer effects by blocking the mevalonate pathway, which is involved in cholesterol production. Statins can also disrupt lipid rafts and caveolae, which can affect cell signaling and survival [22].

Statins inhibit 3-hydroxy-3-methylglutaryl-CoA reductase (HMGCR), which is the enzyme that converts HMG-CoA to mevalonate. More so, statins also reduce cholesterol levels, which can disrupt cell membrane structure, while also suppressing the biosynthesis of geranylgeranyl pyrophosphate (GGPP), which can in turn activate mitochondrial apoptotic signaling pathways, as have been seen with statins inhibiting cell proliferation in vitro and tumor growth in animal models, as well as in some studies that showed a decreased cancer-specific mortality rate in patients who were prescribed statins [23].

Concerning the lipid rafts and caveolae, statins disrupt lipid rafts, which can also affect oncogenic cell signaling, proliferation, and survival. Furthermore, statins can also indirectly affect caveolin-1 (CAV1) and such other related proteins in the micro-domains, leading to CAV1 degradation, altered cell signaling, and apoptosis [24].

Lipid rafts and caveolae as seen in **Figures 4** and **5**, which are specialized, cholesterol-rich micro-domains in the cell membrane, are central to cancer stem cell (CSC) behavior and tumor progression. These structures act as hubs for key signaling pathways like Wnt/β-catenin, Hedgehog, Notch, and TGF-β, all of which drive CSC self-renewal, plasticity, epithelial-mesenchymal transition (EMT), and communication with the tumor microenvironment. Caveolae, a subset of lipid rafts characterized by the protein

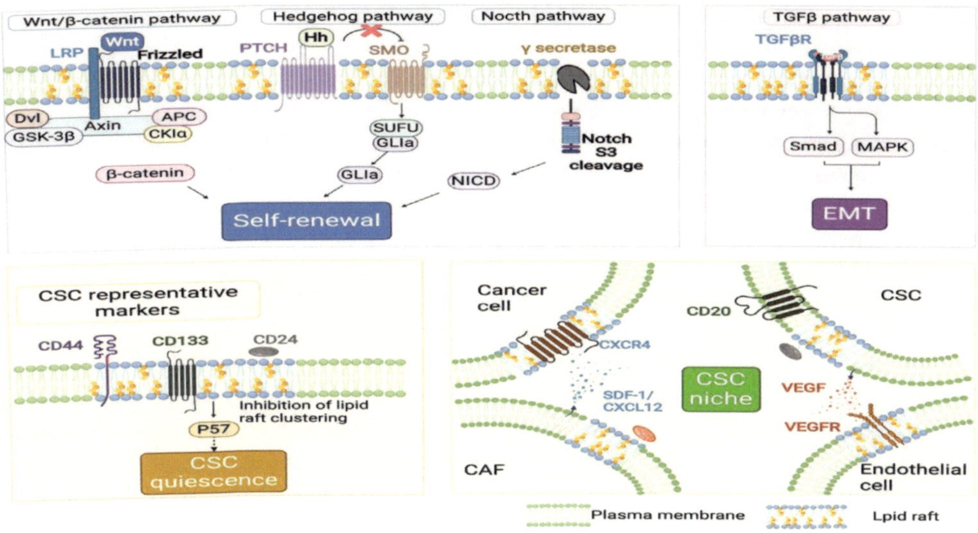

Figure 4.
Lipid rafts in cancer stem cell: A target for statin use in cancer eradication [25]. NICD – Notch Intracellular Domain, CSC – Cancer Stem Cell, KIP – cyclin-dependent Kinase Inhibitor p57.

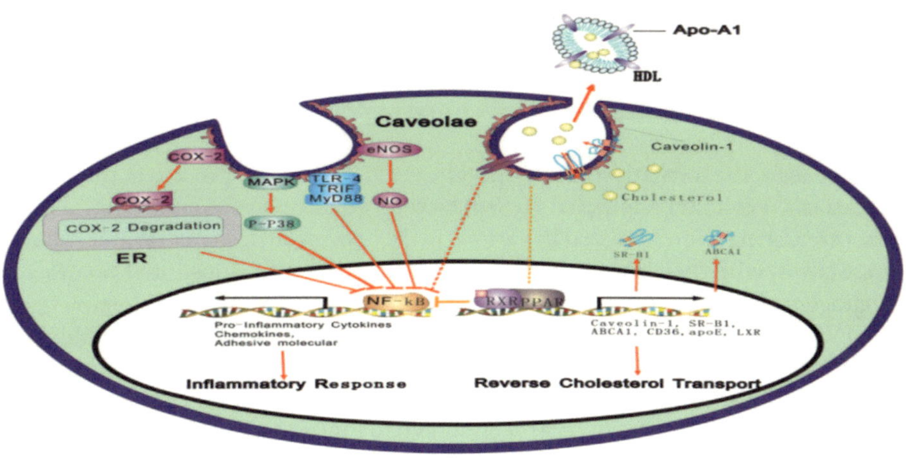

Figure 5.
Role of caveolae in tumorigenesis.

caveolin-1 (CAV1), also contributes to tumorigenesis by regulating endocytosis, growth factor signaling, and cellular adhesion. Overexpression or dysregulation of CAV1 has been linked to tumor cell survival, metastasis, and resistance to therapy. Thus, incorporation of Statins (by inhibiting cholesterol synthesis) disrupts both lipid rafts and caveolae, impairing the organization and function of these signaling domains. This interference weakens oncogenic signaling, impairs CSC survival, and reduces tumor-supportive communication, making cancer cells more vulnerable to treatment [25].

Additionally, statins can also induce autophagy, thus, reducing the viability of tumor cells, and the induction of ferroptosis (a form of programmed cell death), as well as the modulation of angiogenesis, tumor metastasis, and tumor microenvironment [26, 27].

2.1 Targeting oncoproteins and cellular proliferation

Statins, which are primarily known as HMG-CoA reductase inhibitors, exhibit anti-proliferative properties that extend beyond their lipid-lowering effects. By targeting key oncoproteins and cellular pathways, statins interfere with cancer cell proliferation and survival, offering a compelling rationale for their repurposing in oncology [26].

While statins are widely recognized for their ability to reduce total cholesterol and low-density lipoprotein (LDL) levels, they also modestly increase high-density lipoprotein (HDL) levels. These effects contribute to cardiovascular protection, but emerging evidence suggests a parallel role in cancer prevention and therapy. Studies indicate that statins can induce apoptosis in leukemia cells and reduce tumor cell invasion and metastasis, potentially through modulation of the Akt protein signaling pathway. Akt, a serine–threonine kinase within the PI3K pathway, plays a pivotal role in cell proliferation, survival, and metabolism. Its inhibition disrupts key processes critical for cancer cell growth. Statins also up-regulate the tumor suppressor PTEN, which antagonizes PI3K signaling, reducing cancer cell survival and growth [18].

Simvastatin, in particular, has demonstrated the ability to inhibit cyclin-dependent kinase 4 (CDK4) and cyclin D (CyclinD), arresting the cell cycle in the S phase. It also up-regulates CDK inhibitors such as p16 and p27, further halting proliferation. Studies by Sarbassova et al. revealed that simvastatin and atorvastatin regulate signaling molecules such as mTOR, p53, and BCL-2, enhancing their anti-proliferative effects. These molecules are critical in promoting apoptosis and inhibiting cell cycle progression (**Figure 6**) [28].

2.2 Inhibition of angiogenesis in cancer progression

Angiogenesis, the formation of new blood vessels, is a critical process in tumor growth and metastasis. Vascular endothelial growth factor (VEGF) plays a central role in this process, often being overexpressed in various malignancies such as gastric and colorectal cancers. Statins, with their diverse biochemical actions, have demonstrated significant anti-angiogenic potential, which may contribute to their utility in cancer therapy [29].

VEGF is up-regulated in hypoxic tumor environments, driven by hypoxia-inducible factor-1 alpha (HIF-1α). This leads to the proliferation of vascular endothelial cells and the activation of plasminogen activators, facilitating angiogenesis and tumor progression. Statins, particularly simvastatin, have been shown to inhibit VEGF-mediated angiogenesis by blocking the isoprenylation of RhoA, a key protein involved in cellular signaling pathways promoting endothelial cell proliferation [18, 30]. Park et al. [31] demonstrated that simvastatin disrupts VEGF-mediated angiogenesis by targeting RhoA signaling, effectively reducing vascular endothelial cell proliferation and migration.

Thrombospondin-2 (TSP-2), an endogenous angiogenesis inhibitor, is up-regulated by statins in specific cancers [32]. Cerivastatin, for instance, has been shown to promote TSP-2 expression in breast cancer cells, effectively suppressing new blood vessel formation. This highlights a dual mechanism through which statins exert anti-angiogenic effects—by both inhibiting pro-angiogenic factors like VEGF and enhancing the expression of anti-angiogenic mediators like TSP-2 [32, 33].

2.3 Role of statins in inducing apoptosis

The induction of apoptosis, a critical process for eliminating dysfunctional or malignant cells, is a key mechanism through which statins exert anti-cancer effects.

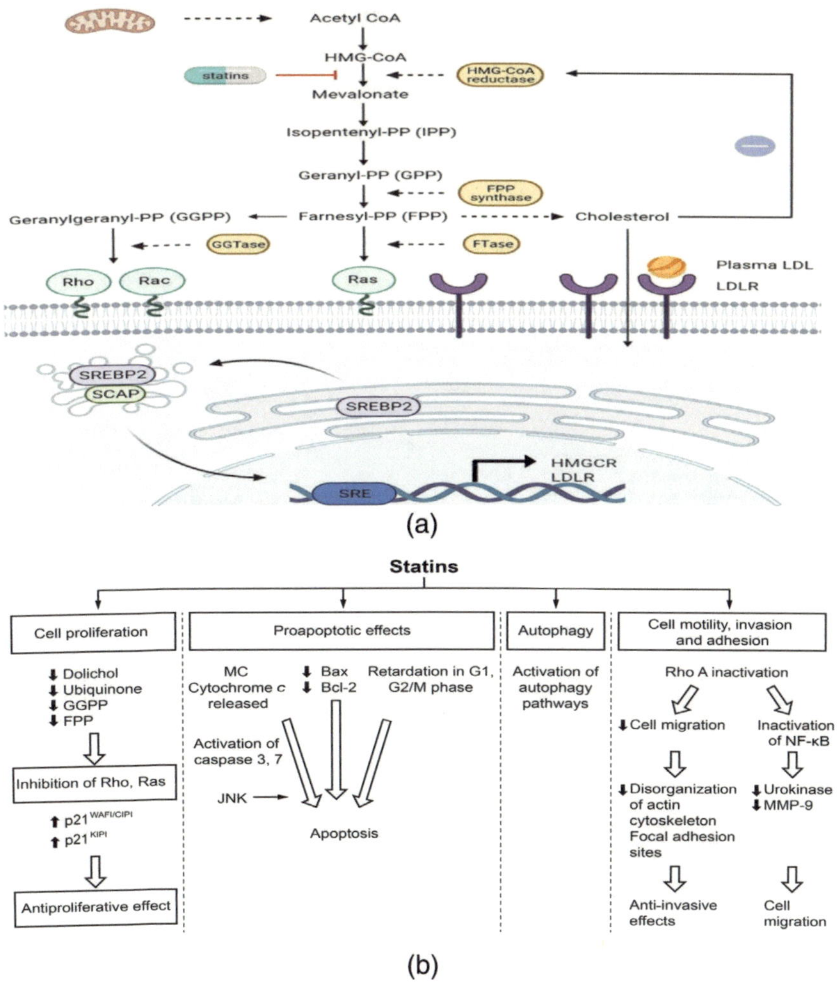

Figure 6.
(A): Importance of statins in blockade of oncoproteins and cellular proliferation [26]. (B): Chart of statins activity against oncoproteins and cellular proliferation [26–28].

Numerous studies have demonstrated that statins can regulate tumor cell apoptosis by interfering with multiple signaling pathways, modulating cell cycle dynamics, and inhibiting the invasive and metastatic capabilities of cancer cells [17, 28].

Statins block the mevalonate pathway by inhibiting HMG-CoA reductase, which is crucial for the synthesis of isoprenoids such as farnesyl pyrophosphate (FPP) and geranylgeranyl pyrophosphate (GGPP). These isoprenoids are required for the post-translational modification and membrane localization of Ras superfamily proteins, which play pivotal roles in several signaling pathways. The reduction in signaling via these pathways disrupts tumor cell proliferation, survival, and metastasis, triggering apoptosis [31].

Survivin, an apoptosis inhibitor overexpressed in many tumors, is associated with disease progression and resistance to therapy. Chang et al. demonstrated that simvastatin reduces Survivin expression in human colon cancer cells, activating p38 mitogen-activated protein kinase (p38MAPK) and inducing p53 phosphorylation. These molecular events culminate in reduced cell viability and enhanced apoptosis, showcasing statins' potential as agents to overcome tumor cell resistance [34].

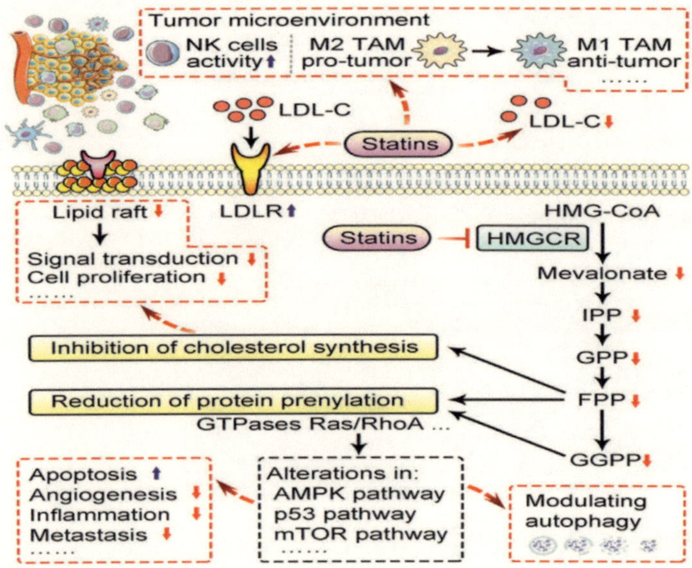

Figure 7.
Multifarious mechanisms of action of statins use in oncology [18, 29–31, 35–40].

2.4 Modulating immune responses in cancer

The tumor microenvironment often features an immunosuppressive state that facilitates tumor progression. Statins have shown promise in modulating immune responses, thereby enhancing the body's ability to combat malignancies [35, 36]. Statins alter the balance of T-helper cell responses through Th1 suppression and Th2 promotion. This shift in T-cell dynamics reduces tumor-promoting inflammation and supports immune-mediated tumor suppression [37].

Statins also inhibit macrophage and microglial production of pro-inflammatory cytokines, reducing tumor-promoting inflammation [38]. Also, by down-regulating the expression of major histocompatibility complex (MHC) class II molecules, CD40, and CD80/CD86 on antigen-presenting cells, statins diminish excessive immune activation, creating a more balanced immune response [39, 40]. **Figure 7** gives insights into the immunomodulatory effects of statins, including their ability to reduce inflammatory cytokines and alter T-cell responses, thus suggesting potential synergy with immune checkpoint inhibitors [37].

3. Organ-specific applications of statins in cancer

3.1 Statins in breast cancer therapy

Breast cancer is the most prevalent malignancy among women globally, with a diverse molecular landscape encompassing hormone receptor-positive, HER2-positive, and triple-negative breast cancer (TNBC) subtypes. Despite advancements in systemic therapies, resistance to treatment and metastatic progression remain significant hurdles. Statins, initially designed for hyperlipidemia management, have demonstrated promising anticancer properties in preclinical and clinical studies, particularly in hormone-responsive malignancies like breast cancer [20]. This section delves into the mechanisms through which statins modulate breast cancer biology, evaluates the evidence supporting their therapeutic potential, and explores their integration into personalized treatment regimens.

Mechanisms of action of statins in breast cancer include:

1. Cholesterol modulation and membrane dynamics: Breast cancer cells exhibit high cholesterol dependency for maintaining membrane fluidity, proliferation, and signaling. Statins inhibit HMG-CoA reductase, reducing intracellular cholesterol levels and disrupting lipid rafts, essential platforms for receptor-mediated signaling pathways, such as EGFR, HER2, and IGF-1R [41, 42].

2. Impact on cellular proliferation: Isoprenoid Inhibition: By blocking the synthesis of farnesyl pyrophosphate and geranylgeranyl pyrophosphate, statins interfere with Ras, Rho, and Rac GTPases, thereby suppressing cell cycle progression and proliferation [43].

   PI3K/Akt/mTOR pathway: Statins down-regulate this pathway, commonly hyper-activated in breast cancer, thereby reducing tumor growth [44].

3. Induction of apoptosis

   Statins promote apoptosis in breast cancer cells by:

   - Activating pro-apoptotic proteins such as Bax and Bad.
   - Down-regulating anti-apoptotic proteins like Bcl-2 and surviving [34].
   - Increasing reactive oxygen species (ROS), leading to mitochondrial membrane destabilization and cytochrome c release [17]

4. Anti-angiogenic effects: Statins inhibit vascular endothelial growth factor (VEGF) expression and angiogenesis, limiting tumor vascularization. They impair endothelial cell proliferation and migration by modulating integrins and matrix metalloproteinases (MMPs) [30].

5. Immunomodulatory activity: Statins enhance anti-tumor immunity by down-regulating immune checkpoint molecules, such as PD-L1, and promoting the activity of cytotoxic T-cells and natural killer (NK) cells [35].

Figure 8 below summarizes the impact of the various mechanisms of action of statins use in the therapeutic management of breast cancer.

3.2 Statins use in specific breast cancer subtypes

1. *Hormone receptor-positive breast cancer*: Estrogen receptor (ER)-positive breast cancer is heavily influenced by cholesterol-derived estrogens [45]. Statins reduce estrogen biosynthesis by depleting cholesterol levels, potentially enhancing the efficacy of endocrine therapies like tamoxifen or aromatase inhibitors. Synergistic effects have also been observed with selective estrogen receptor degraders (SERDs) in preclinical models [41].

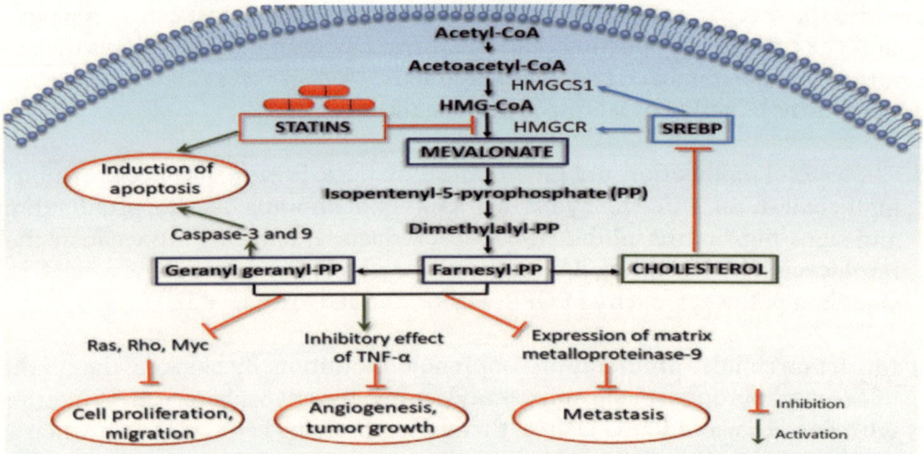

Figure 8.
Mechanisms of action (including inhibition and activation of carcinogenesis with or without statins respectively) in breast cancer (SREBP– Sterol Regulatory Element Binding Protein) [19, 44].

2. *Human epidermal growth factor receptor 2 positive (HER2-Positive) breast cancer*: Statins disrupt HER2 signaling by altering lipid raft composition, leading to receptor internalization and degradation. Preclinical studies indicate enhanced sensitivity to HER2-targeted therapies, such as trastuzumab and lapatinib, when combined with statins [46, 47].

3. *Triple-negative breast cancer (TNBC)*: TNBC is a highly aggressive breast cancer subtype defined by the lack of estrogen receptor (ER), progesterone receptor (PR), and HER2 expression, which limits targeted treatment options. Research indicates that statins may exert therapeutic effects in TNBC by down-regulating cyclin D1, a key cell cycle regulator, and promoting apoptotic cell death in tumor cells [20]. Through epidemiological assessment, observational studies suggest that long-term statin use is associated with reduced breast cancer incidence and improved survival outcomes, and post-diagnosis statin use correlates with lower recurrence rates, particularly in ER-positive and HER2-positive subtypes, especially with the induction of G1-phase cell cycle arrest and apoptosis in breast cancer cells [48].

3.3 Statins in prostate cancer therapy

Prostate cancer is a hormone-dependent malignancy that makes use of androgen receptor signaling, modulation of cholesterol homeostasis, and key cellular pathways for tumor progression, and advancements that have been achieved in its management include androgen deprivation therapy (ADT), chemotherapy, and radiotherapy/ However, the development of resistance and progression to castration-resistant prostate cancer (CRPC) remains a significant clinical challenge. This sub-section explores the mechanisms through which statins may impact prostate cancer progression, evaluates existing evidence, and highlights challenges and opportunities in integrating statins into therapeutic regimens [49].

3.3.1 Mechanisms of action of statins in prostate cancer therapeutic management

Statins in prostate cancer therapeutic management follow the concepts of the prevention of androgen receptor activation (down-regulation of androgen receptor expression and activity), especially with the help of the inhibition of HMG-CoA reductase in cholesterol biosynthesis (by targeting the mevalonate pathway to limit the production of isoprenoids required in post-translational modification of proteins used in androgen receptor signaling) that serves as a precursor for androgen biosynthesis as well, in order to reduce tumor cell proliferation and progression, as well as alteration of composition of lipid rafts in cell membranes that impact signaling and growth pathways, which are also modulated during the induction of autophagic cell death in order to prevent hyperactivation during prostate cancer, and mitogen-activated protein kinase (MAPK), etc., involved in tumor cells proliferation and migration through various pleiotropic effects and inhibition of isoprenoid synthesis [50]; anti-inflammatory effects of statins through the reduction of inflammation-driven prostate tumor progression by inhibiting nuclear factor-kappa B (NF-κB) and cyclooxygenase-2 (COX-2) pathways, thereby enhancing immune surveillance by promoting cytotoxic T-cell activity and reducing the immunosuppressive tumor microenvironment [51, 52]; statins promote programmed cell death by inducing intrinsic apoptosis and autophagy through mitochondrial dysfunction, and they also enhance mitochondrial-mediated apoptosis by increasing pro-apoptotic proteins (e.g., Bcl-2-associated X proteins, Bax, and Bcl-2 antagonist killer, Bak, etc.) and suppressing anti-apoptotic ones like Bcl-2; anti-angiogenic and anti-metastatic effects through inhibition of both VEGF expression and endothelial cell proliferation, thus curtailing the vascular support required for tumor growth and disrupting cell adhesion and migration through the modulation of integrins and matrix metalloproteinases to reduce metastatic potential [53], and through the immunomodulatory effects of statins by reducing programmed death ligand-1 (PD-L1) expression on tumor cells in order to restore T-cell-mediated immunity and promote the activity of natural killer cells and tumor-infiltrating lymphocytes [54].

3.3.2 Statins in prostate cancer subtypes

Prostate cancer can be classified into strategic subtypes. The Gleason Score, illustrated in **Figure 9** and detailed in **Table 1**, grades prostate cancer based on its aggressiveness; higher scores indicate a greater risk of rapid tumor growth and spread, guiding treatment decisions accordingly [56].

A recent 2022 WHO classification mentioned an expanded and more simplified classification to show a better representation of low-grade disease, so as to reduce unnecessary treatment of indolent prostate cancer, especially by using pathological characteristics.

Based on this broad description, most prostate cancers are associated with an increased level of Prostate-Specific Antigen level (PSA), and **Figures 10** and **11** below explain how they are classified according to the types of cellular and genetic compositions involved in cancerous growth, disease progression, as well as possible management strategies.

Additionally, Harshssman et al. conducted a retrospective analysis of 926 prostate cancer patients on androgen deprivation therapy (ADT), and statin users exhibited a significantly longer time to disease progression (27.5 months) compared to non-users (17.4 months), suggesting synergy between statins and ADT [58]. More so, statin use

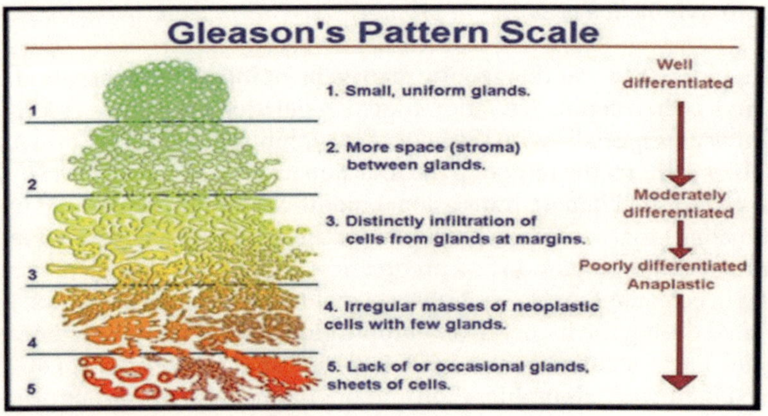

Figure 9.
Gleason's pattern scale [55]. Source: John Murtagh, Jill Rosenblatt, Justin Coleman, Clare Murtagh: John Murtagh's General practice, *7e Copyright © McGraw-Hill Education. All rights reserved.*

Traditional gleason score	New grading system group 1
GLEASON 3 + 3 = 6	GRADE 1
Only individual discrete well-formed glands	
GLEASON 3 + 4 = 7	GRADE 2
Predominantly well-formed glands with a lesser component of poorly-formed/fused/cribriform glands.	
GLEASON 4 + 3 = 7	GRADE 3
Predominantly poorly-formed/fused/cribriform glands with a lesser component of well-formed glands.	
GLEASON 4 + 4 = 8	GRADE 4
Only poorly-formed/fused/cribriform glands or	
• Predominantly well-formed glands with a lesser component lacking or	
• Predominantly lacking glands with a lesser component of well-formed glands.	
GLEASON 9–10	GRADE 5
Lacks gland formation (or with necrosis) with or without poorly-formed/fused/cribriform gland.	
Source: Prostate Conditions Education Council (PCEC).	

Table 1.
Comparing traditional gleason score and new grading system in prostate cancer diagnosis [55].

after diagnosis was associated with a reduction in prostate cancer-specific mortality and a reduction also in all-cause mortality, with the effect more pronounced in patients using lipophilic statins.

3.4 Summary of some clinical trials involving statins in combination cancer therapeutics

Some studies have underscored the effects of statins as valuable player in cancer combination therapies, particularly when combined with conventional or targeted

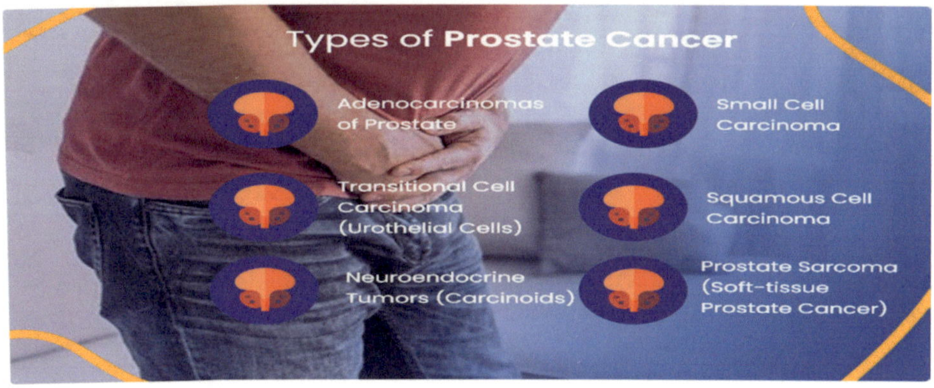

Figure 10.
Types of prostate cancers based on histology and characteristic features [57].

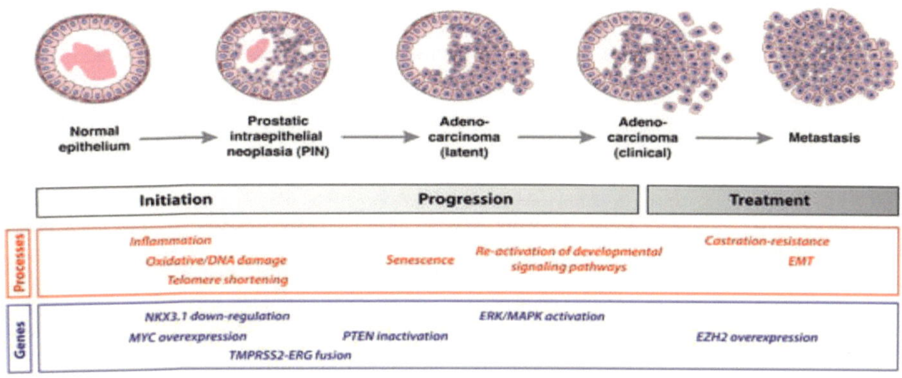

Figure 11.
Genes – Processes association in phases for prostate cancer progression [55].

treatments. **Table 2** has given a summary of some clinical trials involving use of statins in cancer combination therapies and management.

A core mechanism involves inhibition of HMG-CoA reductase, a pivotal enzyme in the mevalonate pathway responsible for producing isoprenoids necessary for protein prenylation. Disruption of this process impairs the activation of proliferative proteins like Ras and Rho and instead favors the up-regulation of pro-apoptotic mediators such as PUMA, as evident in the studies in the studies at the University of California where statins combined with the BCL-2 inhibitor venetoclax led to selective apoptosis in leukemia and lymphoma cells while sparing healthy tissue [67]. Parallel findings in ovarian cancer research, such as those by Zhang et al. [68], demonstrated that statins can enhance the efficacy of PARP inhibitors like niraparib, improving progression-free survival by altering tumor cell viability. Clinical trials—including NCT04418089 (breast cancer), NCT02161822 (colorectal cancer), NCT04776889 (prostate cancer), and NCT00944463 (pancreatic cancer)—provide further evidence of these synergistic effects. In these studies, the integration of statins has been associated with increased sensitivity to chemotherapy, delayed resistance, and enhanced

Cancer type	Trial ID	Combination therapy	Proposed mechanism	Key outcomes
Breast cancer [59]	NCT04705909	Pitavastatin + Neo-adjuvant Chemotherapy	Inhibition of HMG-CoA reductase leading to decreased cyclin D1 and increased caspase-3 levels, promoting apoptosis	Significant tumor size reduction; enhanced response in HER2-positive tumors
Breast cancer [60]	NCT04418089	Simvastatin + CAF (cyclophosphamide, adriamycin, 5-fluorouracil) Chemotherapy	Synergistic effect with doxorubicin; attenuation of ER stress and activation of Akt pathway	Improved clinical response and increased tumor-free surgical margins
Prostate cancer [61]	NCT04026230	Atorvastatin + Androgen Deprivation Therapy (ADT)	Modulation of lipid metabolism; potential delay in castration resistance	Ongoing Phase III trial assessing time to castration resistance and quality of life
Prostate cancer [62]	NCT04776889	Rosuvastatin + ADT	Reprogramming of lipid metabolism; potential enhancement of ADT efficacy	Randomized trial indicating potential benefits in metastatic prostate cancer patients
Lung cancer [63]	NCT01441349	Simvastatin + Irinotecan/Cisplatin	Inhibition of protein prenylation; enhancement of chemotherapy-induced apoptosis	Phase II study showing improved response rates in extensive-disease small cell lung cancer
Hepatocellular carcinoma [64]	NCT03275376	Atorvastatin + Sorafenib	Statins may enhance sorafenib efficacy by modulating tumor cell proliferation and survival pathways	Trial terminated; insufficient data to determine efficacy
Pancreatic cancer	NCT00944463	Simvastatin + Gemcitabine	Statins may sensitize tumor cells to gemcitabine by affecting cell cycle regulation and apoptosis	Trial completed; results pending publication
Locally advanced rectal cancer (LARC) [65]	NCT02161822	Simvastatin + Capecitabine (with concurrent pre-operative concurrent chemo-radiotherapy)	Combined inhibition of MAPK signaling pathway leading to enhanced apoptosis	Simvastatin (80 mg) added to chemo-radiotherapy and capecitabine showed no pCR benefit in LARC but was well tolerated; possible synergy requires further study.

Cancer type	Trial ID	Combination therapy	Proposed mechanism	Key outcomes
Advanced gastric cancer [66]	NCT01099085	Simvastatin + Capecitabine–Cisplatin combination	Statins may improve chemotherapy efficacy by modulating cholesterol metabolism and inducing apoptosis	Clinical trial did not show any increase in the median progression free survival. However, there was no increase in toxicity. More study is required

Table 2.
Summary of some clinical trials involving statins in combination cancer therapies.

apoptotic signaling. Collectively, these insights reflect a growing consensus that statins, beyond their lipid-lowering role, hold significant therapeutic potential in oncology when used as part of a carefully designed combination regimen.

4. Combination therapy with statins: A new horizon

The rationale for incorporating statins into cancer treatment lies in their unique pleiotropic properties. By understanding the multifaceted role of statins in cancer, researchers and clinicians can harness their full potential to improve patient outcomes and expand therapeutic frontiers, affecting key processes, such as cellular proliferation, angiogenesis, and immunomodulation, etc., that cancer cells depend on to thrive. These prompt an increasing emphasis on combination therapies that target multiple pathways simultaneously [69].

4.1 Rationale for combination therapy in cancer treatment

Combination therapy in oncology aims to leverage the distinct and complementary mechanisms of action of multiple agents to enhance therapeutic efficacy while overcoming the limitations of monotherapy. The inclusion of statins in combination regimens for cancer treatment is supported by several compelling rationales, rooted in both their unique biological effects and clinical potential [26].

4.2 Some synergistic effects with conventional therapies

Statins, when combined with standard treatments, can enhance anti-cancer efficacy through complementary mechanisms.

4.2.1 Chemotherapy

a. *Enhanced cytotoxicity and sensitization to chemotherapeutic agents* – Statins sensitize tumors to chemotherapy via tumor microenvironment modification and metabolic disruption [22].

   - *Cisplatin*: Taylor-Harding et al. showed that fluvastatin enhanced cisplatin cytotoxicity in CAOV3 and SKOV3 ovarian cells by disrupting Ras signaling

[70]. Koi et al. also reported lovastatin reversed cisplatin resistance in prostate and cervical cancer via RHOB, KLF2, and KLF6 up-regulation [71]. Similarly, Hu et al. found pitavastatin boosted cisplatin effects in lung cancer (in vitro and in vivo) via Ras/Raf/MEK and PI3K/Akt/mTOR inhibition without added toxicity [72]. Gobel et al. also noted simvastatin with cisplatin increased ovarian cell apoptosis (via cleaved caspase-3 and PARP), and reduced lipid raft formation impaired DNA repair, enhancing cisplatin lethality [73].

- *Doxorubicin*: Mallappa et al. observed that simvastatin suppressed ABCG4-mediated doxorubicin efflux in prostate cancer, increasing drug retention and tumor apoptosis without added toxicity [74]. Kozar et al. demonstrated cerivastatin enhanced doxorubicin and cisplatin activity in breast cancer models [75].

b. *Overcoming chemo-resistance* – Fluvastatin and atorvastatin, combined with doxorubicin, paclitaxel, or topotecan, reduced leukemia proliferation via ERK/MAP kinase inhibition [76]. Simvastatin down-regulated MDR1 and P-gp and this helped in increasing leukemia chemo-sensitivity to drugs and overcoming resistance [77].

- *Inhibition of ABC transporters*: Statins suppress drug efflux proteins like P-gp, increasing intracellular drug levels. They also down-regulate P-gp and COX-2, reducing doxorubicin resistance [78]. Lovastatin also improved Imatinib sensitivity in melanoma by inhibiting ABC transporter efflux [79].

- *5-Fluorouracil (5-FU)*: Statins (such as lovastatin, cerivastatin, and simvastatin) enhanced 5-FU efficacy in colorectal cancer by P-gp inhibition and improved drug retention [80].

- *Modulation of autophagy*: Statins exert anti-cancer effects by modulating autophagy—a process cancer cells use for survival under stress [81]:

    1. Inhibiting HMG-CoA reductase depletes GGPP, activates AMPK, suppresses mTOR, and triggers autophagy [82].

    2. Statins up-regulate p21 via HDAC inhibition or AMPK phosphorylation, causing ER stress and autophagy [83].

    3. They also promote nuclear p53 accumulation, driving autophagic cell death [82].

Sheng et al. demonstrated that in cervical cancer, atorvastatin induced and inhibited autophagy (autophagy-driven anti-tumor activity), reduced tumor growth, and enhanced apoptosis via mevalonate pathway inhibition. Blocking autophagy amplified its cytotoxic effect [84]. As demonstrated in **Figures 12** and **13** below, autophagy regulation is essential to statins' therapeutic action.

4.2.2 Radiotherapy

1. *Radiation sensitization and DNA damage* – Statins can sensitize tumor cells to radiotherapy by augmenting DNA damage and hindering the repair mechanisms that typically protect tumor cells from radiation-induced killing [24].

DOI: http://dx.doi.org/10.5772/intechopen.1012091

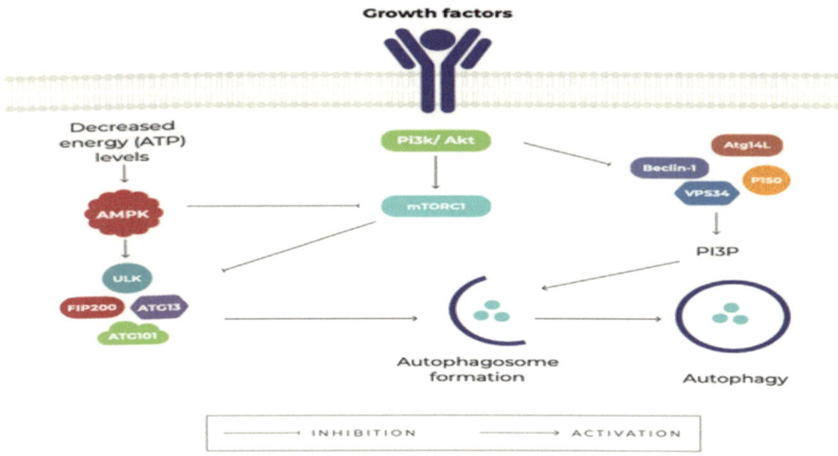

Figure 12.
Mechanisms of action in autophagy process [82, 83].

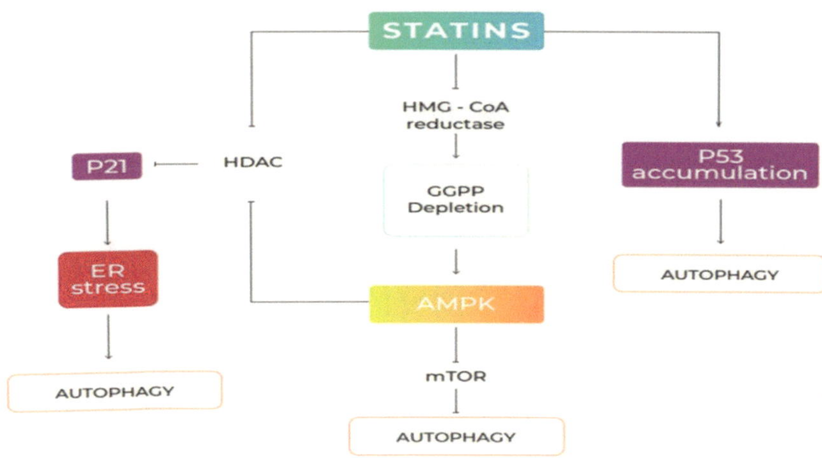

Figure 13.
Impact of statins use in autophagy process in cancer therapies optimization [82, 83].

- *Enhanced DNA damage response*: Statins lower the levels of isoprenoids, which are necessary for the post-translational modification of DNA repair enzymes such as the Rad51 recombinase. This results in defective DNA repair and prolonged DNA damage, increasing the effectiveness of radiotherapy. In prostate cancer models, the combination of radiotherapy and statins (e.g., simvastatin or atorvastatin) caused significant inhibition of tumor growth compared to either treatment alone. A study by Oka et al. investigated the efficacy of combination therapy with statins such as simvastatin and irradiation in androgen-independent prostate cancer cells, as simvastatin altered gene expressions in PC-3 cells in prostate cancer. The combination of simvastatin and irradiation also further enhanced the expression of γH2AX that has been widely reported to be one of the accurate markers of DNA damage in PC-3 cells [85].

- *Increased Reactive Oxygen Species (ROS) production*: Statins elevate intracellular ROS levels, which enhance radiation-induced oxidative stress in tumor cells. Huang et al. identified activation of the cyclic GMP-AMP synthase simulator of the interferon genes (cGAS–STING) pathway in colorectal cancer (HCT116) cells, linking it to increased Type I interferon production and pro-inflammatory signaling [86]. Also, in glioblastoma models, statins further sensitized tumor cells to radiation, as shown by elevated apoptotic markers like cleaved caspase-3 (**Table 3**) [124].

4.3 Targeted therapies

Statins influence several oncogenic pathways and cellular processes that overlap with those targeted by precision therapies, thereby creating opportunities for molecular synergy in targeted therapies. Targeted therapies are designed to interfere with specific molecules driving tumor growth and progression, while statins offer a broader mechanism of action by targeting cholesterol biosynthesis and modulating pleiotropic pathways. The convergence of these targeted therapeutic strategies has the potential to achieve additive or synergistic effects, thus enhancing efficacy by addressing tumor heterogeneity, resistance mechanisms, therapeutic optimization, and overcoming the limitations of monotherapy:

1. *Synergy with tyrosine kinase inhibitors (TKIs)* – Statins enhance the effectiveness of tyrosine kinase inhibitors (TKIs) by disrupting compensatory survival pathways that often undermine the efficacy of TKIs, as seen especially in findings that strongly suggest that combined treatment with other anti-cancer agents may not only provide an enhanced therapeutic response, but also provide a means to avoid toxicity, low bioavailability, or limited therapeutic action associated with high-dose monotherapy [125].

    - *Erlotinib and statins*: Resistance to erlotinib in NSCLC, often due to EGFR T790 mutation, can be overcome by combining it with statins. Simvastatin enhances the anti-proliferative effects of erlotinib by suppressing Akt/mTOR signaling and inducing apoptosis [103]. Similarly, pitavastatin and fluvastatin promote apoptosis, and pitavastatin synergizes with erlotinib to increase cytotoxicity in K-Ras-mutant NSCLC cells [117].

    - *Gefitinib and statins*: Statins like lovastatin enhance gefitinib response in EGFR-mutant and resistant glioblastoma by inhibiting downstream pathways such as Ras/RAF/MAPK, independent of EGFRvIII and PTEN status [87]. In NSCLC with K-Ras mutation, lovastatin and gefitinib together inhibit growth and induce apoptosis via RAF/ERK and Akt pathway down-regulation [89]. Atorvastatin also reverses gefitinib resistance in KRAS-mutant NSCLC, regardless of PIK3CA or PTEN status [120].

2. *mTOR inhibitors* – They are a class of drugs that block the activity of the mammalian target of rapamycin (mTOR), which is a protein kinase involved in cell growth, proliferation, and metabolism, and are also used to treat various diseases, including cancers and auto-immune disorders [126]. Statins can potentiate the effects of mTOR inhibitors such as everolimus through

DOI: http://dx.doi.org/10.5772/intechopen.1012091

Cancer type/Cell line	Statin used	Co-therapy	Dose (μM)	Mechanistic outcome	References
Glioblastoma	Lovastatin	Gefitinib	10	Suppresses Akt pathway signaling	[87]
Human cholangiosarcoma	Lovastatin	Gefitinib	5–10	Enhances TNF-α levels and cell cycle blockade; inhibits LKB1 activation	[88]
Non-small cell lung carcinoma	Lovastatin	Gefitinib	1–5	Promotes apoptosis via increased PARP, caspase-3; down-regulates Bcl-2, RAS, p-RAF, p-ERK1/2, p-AKT, and p-EGFR	[89]
Chronic myeloid leukemia	Lovastatin	Imatinib	5–20	Reduces expression of ABCB1 and ABCG2 efflux transporters	[79]
Gall bladder cancer	Lovastatin	Cisplatin	10–50	Interferes with DNA repair mechanisms	[90]
Prostate cancer	Lovastatin	TRAIL	5	Promotes replication of PRRA, and increases CAR and integrin levels	[91]
Glioblastoma	Lovastatin	Temozolomide	0.625–20	Disrupts autophagic flux	[92]
Anaplastic thyroid cancer	Lovastatin	Troglitazone	1–100	Elevates p21 and p27 expression, inducing G_1 phase arrest	[93]
Prostate cancer	Simvastatin	Docetaxel	25	Enhances Bad levels while reducing Bcl-2, Bcl-xL, cleaved caspase-9/3; stimulates TNF, Fas-L, Traf1, and caspase-8 activity	[94]
Prostate cancer	Simvastatin	Doxorubicin	2.5–20	Down-regulates ABGC4 protein expression	[74]
Malignant	Simvastatin	Doxorubicin	10	Elevates NF-κB activation and nitric oxide production	[95]
Mesothelioma	Mevastatin	Doxorubicin	100		
Colon carcinoma	Simvastatin	5-FU	5 mg/kg	Suppresses Bcl-2, promotes Bax, and reduces tumor angiogenesis	[96]
Human salivary adenoid cystic carcinoma	Simvastatin	MiR-21 inhibitor	1–100	Down-regulates N-cadherin, survivin, and Bcl-2; up-regulates E-cadherin, p53, Bax, and caspase-9	[97]
Pancreatic ductal carcinoma	Simvastatin	Gemcitabine	5–40	Induces Gfi-1 while suppressing CTGF	[98]
Chronic myeloid leukemia	Simvastatin	Imatinib	10–50	Triggers cell cycle arrest; suppresses STAT3 and STAT5 signaling	[99]

Cancer type/Cell line	Statin used	Co-therapy	Dose (μM)	Mechanistic outcome	References
Metastatic melanoma	Simvastatin	Dacarbazine	0.5–1	Lowers RhoA, RhoC, LIM expression; increases p53, p21, p27, caspase-3, and PARP	[100]
Breast cancer	Simvastatin	Pentoxifylline	0.1–50	Promotes autophagy, apoptosis, and cell cycle blockade	[101]
Prostate cancer	Simvastatin	Castration	0.1–20	Facilitates apoptosis and cell cycle arrest via Akt suppression	[102]
Blood cancer	Simvastatin	Ventoclax	5–20	Up-regulates pro-apoptotic proteins p53 and PUMA	[67]
Non-small cell Lung cancer	Simvastatin	Gefitinib, Erlotinib	5	Reduces Akt, β-catenin, survivin, and cyclin D1 expression	[103]
Gastric cancer xenograft	Simvastatin	Capecitabine	10–50	Inhibits NF-κB activity	[104]
Melanoma cells	Simvastatin	5,6-dimethylsanthenone-4-acetic acid	1.5–14	Reduces HIF-α expression	[105]
Breast cancer	Simvastatin	Anti-HER2	1–5	Suppresses YAP/TAZ transcriptional activity	[106]
Colon cancer	Simvastatin + Phenothiazines	Doxorubicin	2.5	Suppresses ABCB1, COX-2, and Bcl-2; boosts Bax expression	[107]
Human myeloid leukemia	Simvastatin, Mevastatin, Lovastatin, Pravastatin	Doxorubicin, Paclitaxel, 5-FU	5–50	Inhibits NF-κB signaling	[78]
Pancreatic cancer	Simvastatin + bisphosphonates	Gemcitabine	0.1–100	Reduces cell viability	[108]
Colon cancer	Simvastatin + Oxicam derivatives	Doxorubicin	5	Up-regulates caspase-3 and Bax; lowers Bcl-2 and COX-2 levels	[109]
Prostate cancer	Simvastatin + Valproic acid	Docetaxel	1–100	Down-regulates YAP signaling	[110]
Acute myeloid leukemia	Fluvastatin	Lestaurtinib (TKI)	0.2–2	Blocks FLT3 protein glycosylation	[111]
HepG2 (Human hepatoma)	Fluvastatin	Trans-activator transcription (TAT) Peptide	1–1000	Induces cell accumulation in pre-G phase	[112]
Melanoma cells	Fluvastatin	Sorafenib	1	Enhances PARP and JNK signaling activity	[113]
Hepatocellular carcinoma	Fluvastatin	Sorafenib	10 mg/kg	Inhibits MAPK and NF-κB signaling pathways	[114]

Cancer type/Cell line	Statin used	Co-therapy	Dose (μM)	Mechanistic outcome	References
Melanoma cells	Fluvastatin	Vemurafenib	1–10	Suppresses Akt expression	[115]
Breast cancer	Fluvastatin, Simvastatin	CH51126766 or Trametinib	0.3	Suppresses Akt, increases PARP cleavage	[116]
Non-small cell Lung cancer	Fluvastatin, Pitavastatin	Erlotinib	100	Induces caspase-3 and PARP activity	[117]
Human osteosarcoma	Fluvastatin, atorvastatin, and simvastatin	Doxorubicin, Cisplatin	10	Reduces MMP-2 expression	[118]
Human cholangiocarcinoma	Atorvastatin	Gemcitabine	5–100	Suppresses Yes-associated protein expression	[119]
Non-small cell lung cancer	Atorvastatin	Gefitinib	1–5	Inhibits both Akt and ERK signaling	[120]
Melanoma cancer	Atorvastatin	Tamoxifen	1–100	Enhances pro-apoptotic Bax and cytochrome C	[121]
Murine mammary adenocarcinoma	Rosuvastatin	Nilotinib	7.5 mg/kg	Activates caspase-3, reduces ERα expression and tumor nitric oxide levels	[122]
Hepatocellular carcinoma	Rosuvastatin	Dasatinib	10, 25, 50	Suppresses phosphorylation of FAK, Src, Ras/Raf, STAT3, Akt; down-regulates HGF, VEGF, MMP-9, Ki67	[123]

Table 3.
Summary of the synergistic action of some statins in combination with anti-cancer drugs to overcome anti-cancer therapy resistance.

complementary molecular mechanisms. Nolting et al. demonstrated that lovastatin, which targets ERK and AKT signaling, enhanced everolimus-induced cytotoxicity across various neuroendocrine and hepatocellular carcinoma cell lines, including GOT, BON1, H727, HepG2, Huh7, MPC, and MTT [127]. This synergy is partly attributed to statins' inhibition of the mevalonate pathway, which depletes isoprenoid intermediates essential for mTOR activation (**Figures 14** and **15**) [26].

Therefore, the mTOR pathway, a central regulator of cell growth, is frequently up-regulated in cancers. While targeted therapies like everolimus inhibit

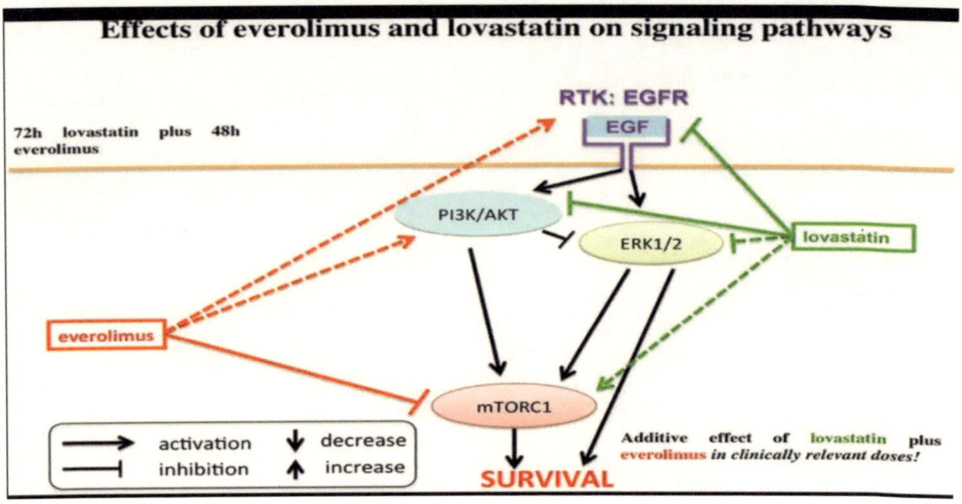

Figure 14.
Effects of everolimus and lovastatin combination on signaling pathways [127].

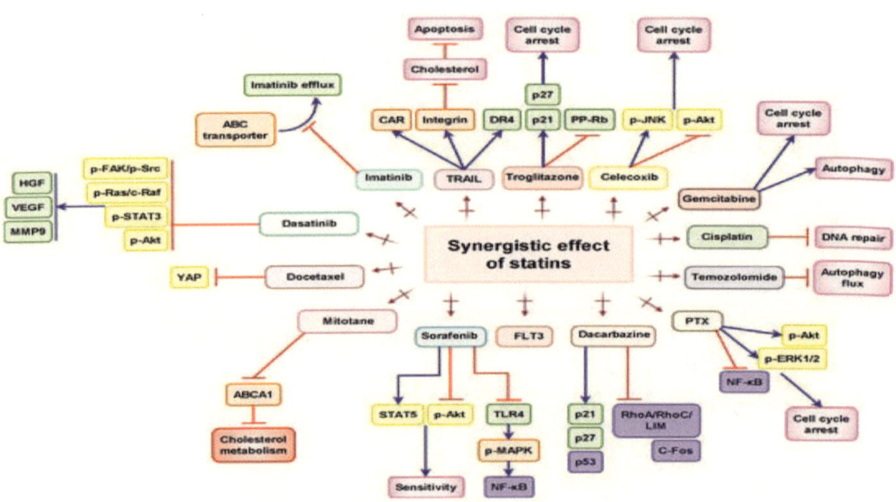

Figure 15.
Overview of the synergistic actions of statins with effects (Blue arrow: Up-regulation, Black line: Inhibition/suppression, Red arrow: Combination of statin with indicated drugs) [69].

mTOR directly, statins enhance this inhibition by down-regulating upstream activators, such as Ras and Akt, through reduced prenylation. This dual blockade of the mTOR pathway results in more profound inhibition of cancer cell proliferation [127].

4.4 Overcoming resistance to targeted therapies

Resistance to targeted therapies is a significant barrier in cancer treatment, often arising from compensatory pathway activation, genetic mutations, or tumor microenvironment changes [26]. By briefly highlighting the points as summarized in **Figure 16** below, statins can address these resistance mechanisms through:

- *Compensatory pathway suppression:* Resistance to RTKIs often involves the activation of alternative pathways, such as PI3K/Akt or STAT3. By inhibiting prenylation, statins block the activation of these alternative pathways, restoring tumor sensitivity to RTKIs [24, 128].

- *Epigenetic modulation*: Emerging evidence such as seen with Lin et al. suggests that statins influence epigenetic regulators, such as histone deacetylases (HDACs) and DNA methyltransferases, which are implicated in therapy resistance [129]. This epigenetic modulation may re-sensitize tumors to targeted therapies.

- *Immunomodulatory effects*: Resistance to immune checkpoint inhibitors, such as anti-PD-1/PD-L1 therapies, is partly driven by an immunosuppressive tumor microenvironment (TME). Mao et al. showed evidence of statins reshaping inflamed tumor microenvironment and enhancing immune checkpoint blockade in non-small cell lung cancer [130]. Statins enhance the efficacy of these therapies by reducing regulatory T cells (Tregs) and myeloid-derived suppressor cells (MDSCs) in the TME, thus promoting anti-tumor immunity, such as seen in the

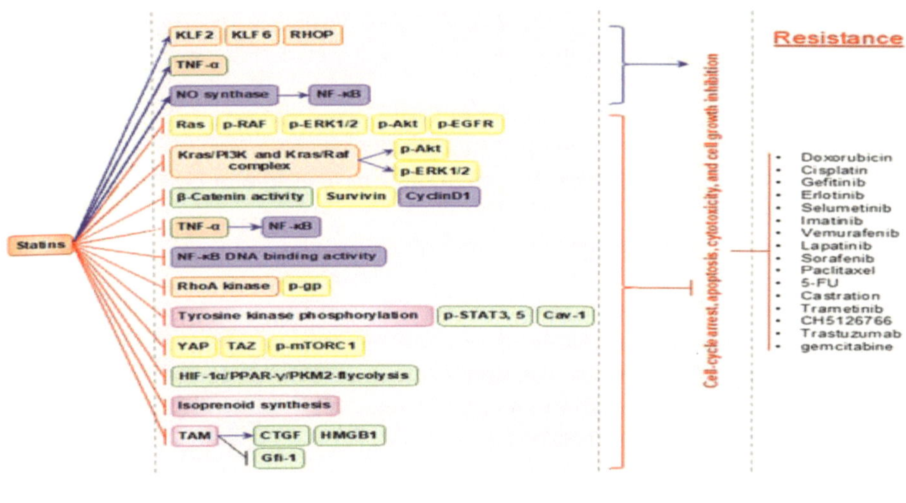

Figure 16.
Statins use in overcoming anti-cancer drug chemo-resistance (Blue arrow: Up-regulation, Red lines: Inhibition/suppression) [69].

research work of Kansal et al. where certain statins medications such as simvastatin, lovastatin, fluvastatin, pitavastatin, atorvastatin, rosuvastatin, and pravastatin) were evaluated to see how they enhance responses to immune checkpoint blockade in head and neck cancer models [131].

5. Advances in statin research for cancer therapy

Statins, traditionally used as lipid-lowering agents, have gained significant attention in oncology due to their pleiotropic effects on cellular processes critical for tumor development and progression [26, 132]. This section delves into the scientific advancements and innovations driving the integration of statins into cancer therapy, highlighting novel mechanisms, preclinical evidence, and translational research, while emphasizing areas for future exploration.

5.1 Unraveling novel mechanisms of action

Recent studies have expanded our understanding of statins' anticancer mechanisms, beyond the inhibition of the mevalonate pathway:

- *Inhibition of cancer stem cells (CSCs)*: Statins have demonstrated efficacy in disrupting CSC populations, which are often responsible for tumor recurrence and metastasis. For example, statins such as atorvastatin and simvastatin have been shown to target CSCs in triple-negative breast cancer by down-regulating the Yes-associated protein (YAP)/TAZ signaling pathway.

- *Epigenetic modulation*: Statins modulate chromatin architecture and gene expression through histone deacetylase inhibition and DNA demethylation, promoting the activation of tumor suppressor genes such as cyclin-dependent kinase inhibitor 2A (CDKN2A) [133].

- *Ferroptosis induction*: Emerging research has revealed statins' ability to induce ferroptosis, an iron-dependent form of programmed cell death, particularly in therapy-resistant cancers like pancreatic adenocarcinoma and glioblastoma [134].

- *Impact on the tumor microenvironment (TME)*: Statins reduce immunosuppressive signals within the TME by lowering myeloid-derived suppressor cells and regulatory T-cells, thereby enhancing the efficacy of immune checkpoint inhibitors [35, 135].

5.2 Challenges and future research directions

The application of statins in oncology, though promising, is not without significant challenges, such as those involving resistance mechanisms, optimizing dosing strategies, addressing safety concerns and adverse effects through the assessment of global health implications, and managing drug–drug interactions among other things. While substantial progress has been made, several challenges remain that require further investigations:

1. *Resistance mechanisms*: Understanding intrinsic and acquired resistance to statins in tumors is critical. Statin resistance may arise from altered cholesterol trans-

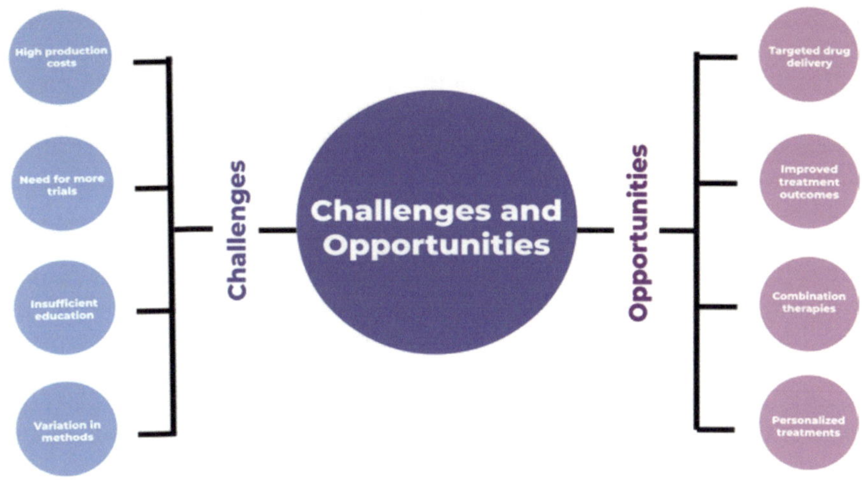
High production costs
Need for more trials
Insufficient education
Variation in methods
Challenges
Challenges and Opportunities
Opportunities
Targeted drug delivery
Improved treatment outcomes
Combination therapies
Personalized treatments

Figure 17.
A summary of the challenges and opportunities in statins use in oncology [136].

port, up-regulation of MDR2 proteins, LDL receptor induction, increased activity of stearoyl-CoA desaturase and HMG-CoA reductase, and genetic polymorphisms affecting metabolism and tolerance.

2. *Dosing strategies*: Determining the optimal statin type, dose, and duration for cancer therapy without compromising safety is a key area of ongoing research.

3. *Cancer type specificity*: While statins show promise in certain cancers (e.g., breast, prostate, and colorectal), their efficacy in others such as seen in melanoma and hepatocellular carcinoma, etc., remains uncertain, thus necessitating further subtype-specific studies.

4. *Global health implications*: Low- and middle-income countries account for nearly 80% of global cancer mortality, a disparity that likely stems from limited access to comprehensive cancer care, including essential pharmacologic treatments, especially in resource-constrained regions. Thus, evaluating statins' cost-effectiveness and accessibility in low- and middle-income countries is essential for broader implementation (**Figure 17**).

5.3 Future outlook and directions: Mechanistic interactions of statins in combination oncology therapeutics

Statins primarily exert their anticancer effects by inhibiting HMG-CoA reductase, a rate-limiting enzyme in the mevalonate pathway. This blockade not only depletes cholesterol but also suppresses the synthesis of isoprenoid intermediates such as farnesyl pyrophosphate (FPP) and geranylgeranyl pyrophosphate (GGPP), crucial for the post-translational modification of signaling proteins like Ras, Rho, and Rac. Disruption of these modifications compromises tumor cell proliferation, survival, and metastatic potential [70].

In chemotherapy, statins enhance drug cytotoxicity through dual mechanisms: by promoting pro-apoptotic signaling (e.g., up-regulation of Bax, down-regulation of Survivin) and by impairing DNA repair processes. Fluvastatin, for example, synergizes with cisplatin in ovarian cancer by inducing G2/M arrest and elevating caspase-3 activity, effects that are reversible with exogenous GGPP supplementation [70]. Similar chemo-sensitization has been observed in cisplatin-resistant prostate and cervical cancers through up-regulation of RHOB (Ras homolog gene family member B involved in regulating cell shape, adhesion, and apoptosis) and KLF (Krüppel-like factor) transcription factors [71, 72].

Radiotherapy combinations leverage statin-induced increases in intracellular reactive oxygen species (ROS), which potentiate radiation-induced DNA damage. In prostate cancer, simvastatin combined with irradiation significantly reduced tumor cell proliferation and decreased RAD51 expression—a DNA repair protein—thereby enhancing γH2AX expression, a biomarker for double-strand breaks [85]. Additionally, mitochondrial dysfunction mediated by statins has been linked to the activation of the cGAS-STING pathway, enhancing immunogenic cell death in colorectal cancer models [86].

Hyperthermia and ferroptosis-based strategies may benefit from statins' oxidative stress induction, mitochondrial destabilization, and disruption of redox homeostasis. These effects, driven by reduced CoQ10 synthesis and ROS accumulation, render cancer cells more vulnerable to heat shock and iron-dependent lipid peroxidation mechanisms [134].

In apoptosis-focused regimens, statins amplify mitochondrial-mediated pathways by altering BCL-2 family protein balance, up-regulating p53-related mediators like PUMA, and enhancing cytochrome c release [82, 86, 89, 97]. Notably, studies from the University of California showed that combining statins with BCL-2 inhibitor venetoclax selectively induced apoptosis in leukemia cells while sparing normal lymphocytes [67].

Immunologically, statins recalibrate the tumor microenvironment by dampening chronic inflammation, altering T-helper cell polarization, and modulating checkpoint molecule expression. They reduce pro-inflammatory cytokines and support anti-tumor T-cell activation, thereby enhancing the efficacy of checkpoint inhibitors [37, 38, 44]. This helps to position statins as promising co-agents in immunotherapy, particularly in "cold" tumors where immune activation is insufficient.

Emerging gene therapy approaches may also benefit from statin-induced changes in membrane fluidity and endocytosis, improving vector delivery and transgene expression. Moreover, the downregulation of lipid raft and caveolae domains—which serve as key platforms for receptor signaling—may suppress oncogenic receptor activation and enhance gene therapy uptake [22–27, 75].

The future of statins in oncology lies in their thoughtful incorporation into rationally designed therapeutic regimens. Clinical trials such as NCT04418089 (breast cancer), NCT04776889 (prostate cancer), and NCT02161822 (colorectal cancer) have demonstrated both safety and potential for synergy in combination settings [71, 72]. However, the full realization of their therapeutic potential requires patient-specific stratification, real-time biomarker monitoring and pharmacogenomic-guided dosing strategies to mitigate toxicity and maximize efficacy [68, 74], to help amplify the therapeutic efficacy of diverse oncologic treatments.

6. Conclusion

Statins, long known for their cardiovascular benefits, have emerged as biologically potent agents in oncology owing to their ability to disrupt critical pathways involved in tumor growth and survival. At the heart of their anticancer potential is the inhibition of HMG-CoA reductase, which impairs the mevalonate pathway—an essential source of isoprenoids required for the post-translational prenylation of small GTPases such as Ras, Rho, and Rac. These proteins orchestrate many oncogenic processes, including proliferation, migration, invasion, and resistance to apoptosis. In parallel, statins alter membrane micro-domains such as lipid rafts and caveolae, destabilizing signaling platforms that cancers rely on for growth and immune evasion. Through these mechanisms, statins influence a wide spectrum of cancer hallmarks, including cell cycle progression, mitochondrial integrity, redox homeostasis, and immune regulation.

In summary, statins occupy a unique niche in oncology at the intersection of metabolism, signaling, and immunity. Their multifaceted mechanisms provide multiple therapeutic entry points, but realizing their full potential will require precision—not only in molecular targeting, but also in trial design, biomarker use, and clinical integration. As our understanding of tumor heterogeneity deepens, statins may well emerge as a cornerstone in tailored, mechanism-based combination cancer therapy.

Author details

Oluwafemi Ajoyemi Ala
University College Hospital, Ibadan, Nigeria

*Address all correspondence to: ala.oluwafemii@gmail.com

References

[1] Endo A. A historical perspective on the discovery of statins. Proceedings of the Japan Academy. Series B, Physical and Biological Sciences. 2010;**86**(5):484-493. DOI: 10.2183/pjab.86.484

[2] Group S.S.S.S. Randomised trial of cholesterol lowering in 4444 patients with coronary heart disease: The Scandinavian simvastatin study (4S). Lancet. 1994;**344**:1383-1389

[3] Istvan ES, Deisenhofer J. Structural mechanism for statin inhibition of HMG-CoA reductase. Science. 2001;**292**:1160-1164

[4] Ziaeian B, Fonarow GC. Statins and the prevention of heart disease. JAMA Cardiology. 2017;**2**:464

[5] Lee SE, Chang HJ, Sung JM, Park HB, Heo R, Rizvi A, et al. Effects of statins on coronary atherosclerotic plaques: The PARADIGM study. JACC: Cardiovascular Imaging. 2018;**11**:1475-1484

[6] Alberts AW, Chen J, Kuron G, Hunt V, Huff J, Hoffman C, et al. Mevinolin: A highly potent competitive inhibitor of hydroxymethylglutaryl-coenzyme a reductase and a cholesterol-lowering agent. Proceedings of the National Academy of Sciences of the United States of America. 1980;**77**:3957-3961

[7] Endo A, Kuroda M, Tsujita Y. ML-236A, ML-236B, and ML-236C, new inhibitors of cholesterogenesis produced by Penicillium citrinum. Journal of Antibiotics. 1976;**29**:1346-1348

[8] Muscoli S, Ifrim M, Russo M, Candido F, Sanseviero A, Milite M, et al. Current options and future perspectives in the treatment of Dyslipidemia. Journal of Clinical Medicine. 2022;**11**:4716

[9] Brown JS, Amend SR, Austin RH, Gatenby RA, Hammarlund EU, Pienta KJ. Updating the definition of cancer. Molecular Cancer Research. 2023;**21**(11):1142-1147. DOI: 10.1158/1541-7786. MCR-23-0411

[10] Okasha S. Cancer and the Levels of Selection. The British Journal for the Philosophy of Science. Cambridge University Press; 2023

[11] Karagiannis AD, Liu M, Toth PP, Zhao S, Agrawal DK, Libby P, et al. Pleiotropic anti-atherosclerotic effects of PCSK9 inhibitors from molecular biology to clinical translation. Current Atherosclerosis Reports. 2018;**20**:20

[12] Zhang Q, Dong J, Yu Z. Pleiotropic use of statins as non-lipid lowering drugs. International Journal of Biological Sciences. 2020;**16**:2704-2711

[13] Morofuji Y, Nakagawa S, Ujifuku K, Fujimoto T, Otsuka K, Niwa M, et al. Beyond lipid-lowering: Effects of statins on cardiovascular and cerebrovascular diseases and cancer. Pharmaceuticals. 2022;**15**:151

[14] Mullen PJ, Yu R. Longo J et al the interplay between cell signaling and the mevalonate pathway in cancer. Nature Reviews. Cancer. 2016;**16**:718-731

[15] Pandyra AA, Mullen PJ. Goard CA et al genome-wide RNAi analysis reveals that simultaneous inhibition of specific mevalonate pathway genes potentiates tumor cell death. Oncotarget. 2015;**6**:26909-26921

[16] Mo H, Elson CE. Studies of the isoprenoid-mediated inhibition of mevalonate synthesis applied to cancer chemotherapy and chemoprevention.

Experimental Biology and Medicine (Maywood, N.J.). 2004;**229**:567-585

[17] Zhu Y, Casey P, Kumar A, et al. Deciphering the signaling networks underlying simvastatin-induced apoptosis in human cancer cells: Evidence for non-canonical activation of RhoA and Rac1 GTPases. Cell Death and Disease. 2013;**4**:e568. DOI: 10.1038/cddis.2013.103

[18] Jiao Z, Cai H, Long Y, Sirka OK, Padmanaban V, Ewald AJ, et al. Statins-induced GGPP depletion blocks macropinocytosis and starves cells with oncogenic defects. Proceedings. National Academy of Sciences. United States of America. 2020;**117**(8):4158-4168. DOI: 10.1073/pnas.1917938117

[19] Breast Cancer Research Foundation. BCRF-Supported Study Discovers Common Cholesterol Medication Starves Cancer Cells. BCRF.org. 2020. Available from: https://www.bcrf.org/blog/study-finds-statins-cholesterol-medication-starves-cancer [Accessed: December 17, 2024]

[20] Nowakowska MK, Lei X, Thompson MT, Shaitelman SF, Wehner MR, Woodward WA, et al. Association of statin use with clinical outcomes in patients with triple-negative breast cancer. Cancer. 2021;**127**(22):4142-4150. DOI: 10.1002/cncr.33797

[21] Di HU. Drug-targeted Mendelian randomized study of the protective effect of statins against breast cancer. Cancer Research on Prevention and Treatment. 2025;**52**(2):165-171. DOI: 10.3971/j.issn.1000-8578.2025.24.0654

[22] Zaky MY, Fan C, Zhang H, Sun XF. Unraveling the anticancer potential of statins: Mechanisms and clinical significance. Cancers (Basel). 2023;**15**(19):4787. DOI: 10.3390/cancers1519487

[23] Fatehi HA. Current perspectives on statins as potential anti-cancer therapeutics: Clinical outcomes and underlying molecular mechanisms. Translational Lung Cancer Research. 2019;**8**(5):692-699. DOI: 10.21037/tlcr.2019.09.08

[24] Ricco N, Kron SJ. Statins in cancer prevention and therapy. Cancers (Basel). 2023;**15**(15):3948. DOI: 10.3390/cancers15153948

[25] Zhang S, Zhu N, Li HF, et al. The lipid rafts in cancer stem cell: A target to eradicate cancer. Stem Cell Research & Therapy. 2022;**13**:432. DOI: 10.1186/s13287-022-03111-8

[26] Jiang W, Hu JW, He XR, et al. Statins: A repurposed drug to fight cancer. Journal of Experimental & Clinical Cancer Research. 2021;**40**:241. DOI: 10.1186/s13046-021-02041-2

[27] Chengyu L, Bicheng H, Hong C, Jiajian S, Yuchen C, Kun H. New insights into the therapeutic potentials of statins in cancer. Frontiers in Pharmacology. 2023;**14**:1663-9812. DOI: 10.3389/fphar.2023.1188926

[28] Sarbassova G, Nurlan N, Al Shammari BR, Francis N, Alshammari M, Aljofan M. Investigating potential anti-proliferative activity of different statins against five cancer cell lines. Saudi Pharmaceutical Journal. 2023;**31**(5):727-735. DOI: 10.1016/j.jsps.2023.03.013

[29] Relja B, Meder F, Wilhelm K, Henrich D, Marzi I, Lehnert M. Simvastatin inhibits cell growth and induces apoptosis and G0/G1 cell cycle arrest in hepatic cancer cells. International Journal of Molecular Medicine. 2010;**26**(5):735-741. DOI: 10.3892/ijmm_00000520

[30] Takenaka M, Hirade K, Tanabe K, Akamatsu S, Dohi S, Matsuno H, et al. Simvastatin stimulates VEGF release via p44/p42 MAP kinase in vascular smooth muscle cells. Biochemical and Biophysical Research Communications. 2003;**301**:198-203. DOI: 10.1016/s0006-291x(02)03014-0

[31] Park HJ, Kong D, Iruela-Arispe L, Begley U, Tang D, Galper JB. 3-Hydroxy-3-Methylglutaryl coenzyme a reductase by inhibiting the geranylgeranylation of RhoA. Circulation Research. 2002;**91**(2):143-150. DOI: 10.1161/01.res.0000028149.15986.4c

[32] Streit M, Riccardi L, Velasco P, Brown LF, Hawighorst T, Bornstein P, et al. Thrombospondin-2: A potent endogenous inhibitor of tumor growth and angiogenesis. Proceedings of the National Academy of Sciences of the United States of America. 1999;**96**(26):14888-14893. DOI: 10.1073/pnas.96.26.14888

[33] Denoyelle C, Vasse M, Korner M, Mishal Z, Ganne F, Vannier JP, et al. Cerivastatin, an inhibitor of HMG-CoA reductase, inhibits the signaling pathways involved in the invasiveness and metastatic properties of highly invasive breast cancer cell lines: An in vitro study. Carcinogenesis. 2001;**22**:1139-1148. DOI: 10.1093/carcin/22.8.1139

[34] Chang HL, Chen CY, Hsu YF, Kuo WS, Ou G, Chiu PT, et al. Simvastatin induced HCT116 colorectal cancer cell apoptosis through p38MAPK-p53-survivin signaling cascade. Biochimica et Biophysica Acta (BBA) - General Subjects. 2013;**1830**(8):4053-4064. DOI: 10.1016/j.bbagen.2013.04.011

[35] Kwak B, Mulhaupt F, Myit S, Mach F. Statins as a newly recognized type of immunomodulator. Nature Medicine. 2000;**6**:1399-1402. DOI: 10.1038/82219

[36] Sivakumar B, Harry LE, Paleolog EM. Modulating angiogenesis: More vs less. Journal of the American Medical Association. 2004;**292**:972-977. DOI: 10.1001/jama.292.8.972

[37] William C, Sek CC. Effect of atorvastatin on Th1 and Th2 cytokine secreting cells during T cell activation and differentiation. Atherosclerosis. 2006;**186**(2):302-309. DOI: 10.1016/j.atherosclerosis.2005.08.013

[38] Dulak J, Józkowicz A. Anti-angiogenic and anti-inflammatory effects of statins: Relevance to anti-cancer therapy. Current Cancer Drug Targets. 2005;**5**(8):579-594. DOI: 10.2174/156800905774932824

[39] Wagner AH, Gebauer M, Guldenzoph B, Hecker M. 3-hydroxyl-3-methylglutaryl coenzyme a reductase-independent inhibition of CD40 expression by atorvastatin in human endothelial cells. Arteriosclerosis, Thrombosis, and Vascular Biology. 2002;**22**:1784-1789

[40] Forero-Pena DA, Gutierrez FRS. Statins as modulators of regulatory T-cell biology. Mediators of Inflammation. 2013;**2013**:167086

[41] Simigdala N, Gao Q. Pancholi S et al cholesterol biosynthesis pathway as a novel mechanism of resistance to estrogen deprivation in estrogen receptor-positive breast cancer. Breast Cancer Research. 2016;**18**:58

[42] Bjarnadottir O, Romero Q. Bendahl PO et al targeting HMG-CoA reductase with statins in a window-of-opportunity breast cancer trial. Breast Cancer Research and Treatment. 2013;**138**:499-508

[43] Graaf MR, Richel DJ, van Noorden CJ, Guchelaar HJ. Effects of statins and farnesyltransferase inhibitors on the development and progression of cancer. Cancer Treatment Reviews. 2004;**30**:609-641. DOI: 10.1016/j.ctrv.2004.06.010

[44] Tsubaki M, Yamazoe Y, Yanae M, Satou T, Itoh T, Kaneko J, et al. Blockade of the Ras/MEK/ERK and Ras/PI3K/Akt pathways by statins reduces the expression of bFGF, HGF, and TGF-β as angiogenic factors in mouse osteosarcoma. Cytokine. 2011;**54**(1):100-107. DOI: 10.1016/j.cyto.2011.01.005

[45] Warner M, Gustafsson JA. On estrogen, cholesterol metabolism, and breast cancer. The New England Journal of Medicine. 2014;**370**:572-573

[46] Wang X, Wang L, Yu Q, Liu Z, Li C, Wang F, et al. The effectiveness of Lapatinib in HER2-positive metastatic breast cancer patients Pretreated with multiline anti-HER2 treatment: A retrospective study in China. Technology in Cancer Research & Treatment. 2021;**Jan-Dec;20**:15330338211037812. DOI: 10/1177/15330338211037812

[47] Calvillo-Arguelles O, Abdel-Qadir H, Michalowska M, Billia F, Suntheralingam S, Amir E, et al. Cardioprotective effects of statins in patients with HER2-positive breast cancer receiving Trastuzumab therapy. The Canadian Journal of Cardiology. 2019;**35**(2):153-159. DOI: 10.1016/cjca.2018.11.028

[48] Wolfe AR, Debeb BG, Lacerda L, Larson R, Bambhroliya A, Huang X, et al. Simvastatin prevents triple-negative breast cancer metastasis in pre-clinical models through regulation of FOXO3a. Breast Cancer Research and Treatment. 2015;**154**(3):495-508. DOI: 10.1007/s10549-015-3645-3

[49] Leslie SW, Soon-Sutton TL, Skelton WP. Prostate cancer. In: StatPearls [Internet]. Treasure Island (FL): StatPearls Publishing; 2025. Available from: https://www.ncbi.nlm.nih.gov/books/NBK470550/ [Accessed: October 4, 2024]

[50] Huang K, Han Y, Chen Y, et al. Tumor metabolic regulators: Key drivers of metabolic reprogramming and the promising targets in cancer therapy. Molecular Cancer. 2025;**24**:7. DOI: 10.1186/s12943-024-02205-6

[51] Nigam M, Mishra AP, Tiwari V, et al. Evaluation of the association of chronic inflammation and cancer: Insights and implications. Biomedicine and Pharmacotherapy. 2023;**164**:115015. DOI: 10.1016/j.biopha.2023.115015

[52] Zhao H, Wu L, Yan G, Chen Y, Zhou M, Wu Y, et al. Inflammation and tumor progression: Signaling pathways and targeted intervention. Signal Transduction and Targeted Therapy. 2021;**6**(1):263. DOI: 10.1038/s41392-021-00658-5

[53] Wong B, Lumma WC, Smith AM, Sisko JT, Wright SD, Cai TQ. Statins suppress THP-1 cell migration and secretion of matrix metalloproteinase 9 by inhibiting geranylgeranylation. Journal of Leukocyte Biology. 2001;**69**:959-962

[54] Han Y, Liu D, Li L. PD-1/PD-L1 pathway: Current researches in cancer. American Journal of Cancer Research. 2020;**10**(3):727-742

[55] Wilt TJ, Brawer MK, Jones KM, Barry MJ, Aronson WJ, Fox S, et al. Prostate cancer intervention versus observation trial (PIVOT) study group. Radical prostatectomy versus observation for localized prostate cancer. The New England Journal of Medicine. 2012;**367**(3):203-213

[56] Wasinger G, Oszwald A, Shariat SF, Comperat E. Histological patterns, subtypes and aspects of prostate cancer: Different aspects, different outcomes. Current Opinion in Urology. 2022;**32**(6):643-648. DOI: 10.1097/MOU.0000000000001038

[57] Sekhoacha M, Riet K, Motloung P, Gumenku L, Adegoke A, Mashele S. Prostate cancer review: Genetics, diagnosis, treatment options, and alternative approaches. Molecules. 2022;**27**(17):5730. DOI: 10.3390/molecules27175730

[58] Harshssman LC, Wang X, Nakabayashi M, Xie W, Valenca L, Werner L, et al. Statin use at the time of initiation of androgen deprivation therapy and time to progression in patients with hormone-sensitive prostate cancer. JAMA Oncology. 2015;**1**(4):495-504. DOI: 10.1001/jamaoncol.2015.2075

[59] Dewidar SA, Hamdy O, Eltantawy A, El-Mesery M, El Gayar AM, Soliman MM. Effect of concomitant use of pitavastatin with neoadjuvant chemotherapy protocols in breast cancer patients: A randomized controlled clinical trial. The Saudi Pharmaceutical Journal. 2022;**30**(10):1486-1496. DOI: 10.1016/j.jsps.2022.07.011

[60] Yulian ED, Siregar NCB. Combination of simvastatin and FAC improves response to neoadjuvant chemotherapy in locally advanced breast cancer. Cancer Research and Treatment. 2021;**53**(4):1072-1083. DOI: 10.4143/crt.2020.1024

[61] Siltari A, Riikonen J, Koskimäki J, Pakarainen T, Ettala O, Boström P, et al. Randomised double-blind phase 3 clinical study testing impact of atorvastatin on prostate cancer progression after initiation of androgen deprivation therapy: Study protocol. BMJ Open. 2022;**12**(4):e050264. DOI: 10.1136/bmjopen-2021-050264

[62] Karkeet RM, Zekri AN, Sayed-Ahmed MM, Sherif GM, Salem SE, Abdelbary A, et al. The prognosis of lipid reprogramming with the HMG-CoA reductase inhibitor, rosuvastatin, in castrated Egyptian prostate cancer patients: Randomized trial. PLoS One. 2022;**17**(12):e0278282. DOI: 10.1371/journal.pone.0278282

[63] Lee Y, Lee SH, Lee GK, Lim EJ, Han JY. A randomized phase II study of irinotecan plus cisplatin with or without simvastatin in ever-smokers with extended disease Small cell lung cancer. Cancer Research and Treatment. 2023;**55**(3):885-893. DOI: 10.4143/crt.2023.283

[64] Wang J, Liu C, Hu R, Wu L, Li C. Statin therapy: A potential adjuvant to immunotherapies in hepatocellular carcinoma. Frontiers in Pharmacology. 2024;**1**(15):1324140. DOI: 10.3389/fphar.2024.1324140

[65] Jo H, Kim ST, Lee J, Park SH, Park JO, Park YS, et al. A phase II study of preoperative chemoradiotherapy with capecitabine plus simvastatin in patients with locally advanced rectal cancer. Cancer Research and Treatment. 2023;**55**(1):189-195. DOI: 10.4143/crt.2021.1527

[66] Kim ST, Kang JH, Lee J, Park SH, Park JO, Park YS, et al. Simvastatin plus capecitabine-cisp109 NN – F latin versus placebo plus capecitabine-cisplatin in patients with previously untreated advanced gastric cancer: A double-blind randomised phase 3 study. European Journal of Cancer. 2014;**50**(16):2822-2830. DOI: 10.1016/j.ejca.2014.08.005

[67] Lee JS, Roberts A, Juarez D, Vo TT, Bhatt S, Herzog LO, et al. Statins enhance the efficacy of venetoclax in blood

cancers. Science Translational Medicine. 2018;**10**(445):eaaq1240. DOI: 10.1126/scitranslmed.aaq1240

[68] Zhang H, Rutkowska A, González-Martín A, Mirza MR, Monk BJ, Vergote I, et al. Potential synergistic effect between niraparib and statins in ovarian cancer clinical trials. Cancer Research Communications. 2024;**5**(1):178-186. DOI: 10.1158/2767-9764.CRC-24-0191

[69] Tilija PN, Jeong CH. Statin as a potential chemotherapeutic agent: Current updates as a monotherapy, combination therapy, and treatment for anti-cancer drug resistance. Pharmaceuticals (Basel). 2021;**14**(5):470. DOI: 10.3390/ph14050470

[70] Taylor HB, Orsulic S, Karlan BY, Li AJ. Fluvastatin and cisplatin demonstrate synergistic cytotoxicity in epithelial ovarian cancer cells. Gynecologic Oncology. 2010;**119**(3):549-556. DOI: 10.1016/j.ygyno.2010.08.017

[71] Koi C, Izumi H, Kurita T, Nguyen TT, Murakami M, Yoshiura Y, et al. Lovastatin induced Kruppel like factor 2 (KLF2), Kruppel like factor 6 (KLF6) and Ras homolog family member B (RHOB) genes and preferentially led to viability reduction of cisplatin-resistant cells. Oncotarget. 2017;**8**:106429-106442

[72] Hu T, Shen H, Huang H, Yang Z, Zhou Y, Zhao G. Cholesterol-lowering drug pitavastatin targets lung cancer and angiogenesis via suppressing prenylation-dependent Ras/Akt/Mtor signaling. Anti-Cancer Drugs. 2020;**31**:377-384

[73] Gobel A, Zinna VM, Dell' Endice S, Jaschke N, Kuhlmann JD, Wimberger P, et al. Anti-tumor effects of mevalonate pathway inhibition in ovarian cancer. BMC Cancer. 2020;**20**(1):703. DOI: 10.1186/s12885-020-07164-x

[74] Mallappa S, Neeli PK, Karnewar S, Kotamraju S. Doxorubicin induces prostate cancer drug resistance by up-regulation of ABCG4 through GSH depletion and CERB activation: Relevance of statins in chemosensitization. Molecular Carcinogenesis. 2019;**58**:1118-1133

[75] Kozar K, Kaminski R, Legat M, Kopec M, Nowis D, Skierski JS, et al. Cerivastatin demonstrates enhanced antitumor activity against human breast cancer cell lines when used in combination doxorubicin or cisplatin. International Journal of Oncology. 2004;**24**:1149-1157

[76] Henslee AB, Steele TA. Combination statin and chemotherapy inhibits proliferation and cytotoxicity of an aggressive natural killer cell leukemia. Biomarker Research. 2018;**6**:26

[77] Zhang XH, Zhang R, Zhu ZL, Xu SN, Li YF. Effects of simvastatin on expression of multidrug resistance gene and Protein of SHI-1 cells. Zhongguo Shi Yan Xue Ye Xue Za Zhi. 2016;**24**:1659-1664

[78] Sroda-Pomianek K, Michalak K, Palko-Labuz A, Uryga A, Swiatek P, Majkowski M, et al. The combined use of Phenothiazines and statins strongly affects doxorubicin-resistance, apoptosis, and cox-2 activity in colon cancer cells. International Journal of Molecular Sciences. 2019;**20**:955

[79] Glodkowska-Mrowka E, Mrowka P, Basak GW, Niesiobedzka-Krezel J, Seferynska I, Wlodarski PK, et al. Statins inhibit ABCB1 and ABCG2 drug transporter activity in chronic myeloid leukemia cells and potentiate anti-leukemic effects of imatinib. Experimental Hematology. 2014;**42**:439-447

[80] Peters GJ, Lankelma J, Kok RM, Noordhuis P, van Groeningen CJ, van der Wilt CL, et al. Prolonged retention of high concentrations of 5-fluorouracil in human and murine tumors as compared with plasma. Cancer Chemotherapy and Pharmacology. 1993;**31**:269-276

[81] Ashrafizadeh M, Ahmadi Z, Farkhondeh T, Samarghandian S. Modulatory effects of statins on the autophagy-therapeutic perspective. Journal of Cellular Physiology. 2019;**235**:3157-3168

[82] Ghavami S, Mutawe MM, Sharma P, Yeganeh B, McNeill KD, Klonisch T, et al. Mevalonate Cascade regulation of airway mesenchymal cell autophagy and apoptosis: A dual role for p53. PLoS One. 2011;**6**:e16523

[83] Yang PM, Chen CC. Life or death? Autophagy in anticancer therapies with statins and histone deacetylase inhibitors. Autophagy. 2011;7:107-108

[84] Sheng B, Song Y, Zhang J, Li R, Wang Z, Zhu X. Atorvastatin suppresses the progression of cervical cancer via regulation of autophagy. American Journal of Translational Research. 2020;**12**:5252-5268

[85] Oka D, Sekine Y, Tsuji Y, Nakayama H, Miyazawa Y, Arai S, et al. Simvastatin enhances the Radio-sensitivity of Androgen-independent Prostate Cancer Cells via inhibition of RAD51 expression. Anticancer Research. 2024;**44**(1):93-98. DOI: 10.21873/anticanres.16791

[86] Huang X, Liang N, Zhang F, Lin W, Ma W. Lovastatin-induced mitochondrial oxidative stress leads to the release of mtDNA to promote apoptosis by activating cGAS-TING pathway in human colorectal cancer cells. Antioxidants (Basel). 2024;**13**(6):679. DOI: 10.3390/antiox13060679

[87] Cemeus C, Zhao TT, Barrett GM, Lorimer IA, Dimitroulakos J. Lovastatin enhances gefitinib activity in glioblastoma cells irrespective of EGFRvIII and PTEN status. Journal of Neuro-Oncology. 2008;**90**:9-17

[88] Yang SH, Lin HY, Chang VH, Chen CC, Liu YR, Wang J, et al. Lovastatin overcomes gefitinib resistance through TNF-α signaling in human cholangiocarcinomas with different LKB1 statuses in vitro and in vivo. Oncotarget. 2015;**6**:23857-23873

[89] Park IH, Kim JY, Jung JI, Han JY. Lovastatin overcomes gefitinib resistance in human non-small cell lung cancer cells with K-Ras mutations. Investigational New Drugs. 2010;**28**:791-799

[90] Zhang Y, Liu Y, Duan J, Wang H, Zhang Y, Qiao K, et al. Cholesterol depletion sensitizes gallbladder cancer to cisplatin by impairing DNA damage response. Cell Cycle. 2019;**18**:3337-3350

[91] Liu Y, Chen L, Gong Z, Shen L, Kao C, Hock JM, et al. Lovastatin enhances adenovirus-mediated TRAIL induced apoptosis by depleting cholesterol of lipid rafts and affecting CAR and death receptor expression of prostate cancer cells. Oncotarget. 2015;**6**:3055-3070

[92] Zhu Z, Zhang P, Li N, Kiang KMY, Cheng SY, Wong VK, et al. Lovastatin enhances cytotoxicity of Temozolomide via impairing Autophagic flux in glioblastoma cells. BioMed Research International. 2019;**2019**:2710693

[93] Zhong WB, Tsai YC, Chin LH, Tseng JH, Tang LW, Horng S, et al. A synergistic anti-cancer effect of Troglitazone and lovastatin in a human anaplastic thyroid cancer cell line and in a mouse xenograft model. International

Journal of Molecular Sciences. 1834;**2018**:19

[94] Goc A, Kochuparambil ST, Al-Husein B, Al-Azayzih A, Mohammad S, Somanath PR. Simultaneous modulation of the intrinsic and extrinsic pathways by simvastatin in mediating prostate cancer cell apoptosis. BMC Cancer. 2012;**12**:409

[95] Riganti C, Orecchia S, Pescarmona G, Betta PG, Ghigo D, Bosia A. Statins revert doxorubicin resistance via nitric oxide in malignant mesothelioma. International Journal of Cancer. 2006;**119**:17-27

[96] Luput L, Sesarman A, Porfire A, Achim M, Muntean D, Casian T, et al. Liposomal simvastatin sensitizes C26 murine colon carcinoma to the antitumor effects of liposomal 5-fluorouracil in vivo. Cancer Science. 2020;**111**:1344-1356

[97] Wang C, Li T, Yan F, Cai W, Zheng J, Jiang X, et al. Effect of simvastatin and microRNA-21 inhibitor on metastasis and progression of human salivary adenoid cystic carcinoma. Biomedicine & Pharmacotherapy. 2018;**105**:1054-1061

[98] Xian G, Zhao J, Qin C, Zhang Z, Lin Y, Su Z. Simvastatin attenuates macrophage-mediated gemcitabine resistance of pancreatic ductal adenocarcinoma by regulating the TGF-β1/Gfi-1 axis. Cancer Letters. 2017;**385**:65-74

[99] Oh B, Kim TY, Min HJ, Kim M, Kang MS, Huh JY, et al. Synergistic killing effect of imatinib and simvastatin on imatinib-resistant chronic myelogenous leukemia cells. Anti-Cancer Drugs. 2013;**24**:20-31

[100] Tsubaki M, Takeda T, Obata N, Kawashima K, Tabata M, Imano M, et al. Combination therapy with dacarbazine and statins improved the survival rate in mice with metastatic melanoma. Journal of Cellular Physiology. 2019;**234**:17975-17989

[101] Castellanos-Esparza YC, Wu S, Huang L, Buquet C, Shen R, Sanchez-Gonzalez B, et al. Synergistic promoting effects of pentoxifylline and simvastatin on the apoptosis of triple-negative MDA-MB-231 breast cancer cells. International Journal of Oncology. 2018;**52**:1246-1254

[102] Ingersoll MA, Miller DR, Martinez O, Wakefield CB, Hsieh KC, Simha MV, et al. Statin derivatives as therapeutic agents for castration-resistant prostate cancer. Cancer Letters. 2016;**383**:94-105

[103] Hwang KE, Kwon SJ, Kim YS, Park DS, Kim BR, Yoon KH, et al. Effect of simvastatin on the resistance to EGFR tyrosine kinase inhibitors in a non-small cell lung cancer with the T790M mutation of EGFR. Experimental Cell Research. 2014;**323**:288-296

[104] Manu KA, Shanmugam MK, Li F, Chen L, Siveen KS, Ahn KS, et al. Simvastatin sensitizes human gastric cancer xenograft in nude mice to capecitabine by suppressing nuclear factor-kappa B-regulated gene products. Journal of Molecular Medicine. 2014;**92**:267-276

[105] Rauca VF, Licarete E, Luput L, Sesarman A, Patras L, Bulzu P, et al. Combination therapy of simvastatin and 5, 6-dimethylxanthenone-4-acetic acid synergistically suppresses the aggressiveness of B16.F10 melanoma cells. PLoS One. 2018;**13**:e0202827

[106] Sethunath V, Hu H, de Angelis C, Veeraraghavan J, Qin L, Wang N, et al. Targeting the mevalonate pathway to

overcome acquired anti-HER2 treatment resistance in breast cancer. Molecular Cancer Research. 2019;**17**:2318-2330

[107] Ahn KS, Sethi G, Aggarwal BB. Reversal of chemoresistance and enhancement of apoptosis by statins through down-regulation of the NF-kappa B pathway. Biochemical Pharmacology. 2008;**75**:907-913

[108] Kawashiri T, Tokunaga A, Kobayashi D, Shimazoe T. Anti-tumor activities of 3-Hydroxy-3-methylglutaryl coenzyme a (HMG-CoA) reductase inhibitors and bisphosphonates in pancreatic cell lines which show poor responses to gemcitabine. Biological & Pharmaceutical Bulletin. 2020;**43**:49-52

[109] Środa-Pomianek K, Michalak K, Palko-Łabuz A, Uryga A, Szczęśniak-Sięga B, Wesołowska O. Simvastatin strongly augments Proapoptotic, anti-inflammatory and cytotoxic activity of Oxicam derivatives in doxorubicin-resistant colon cancer cells. Anticancer Research. 2019;**39**:727-734

[110] Iannelli F, Roca MS, Lombardi R, Ciardiello C, Grumetti L, de Rienzo S, et al. Synergistic antitumor interaction of valproic acid and simvastatin sensitizes prostate cancer to docetaxel by targeting CSCs compartment via YAP inhibition. Journal of Experimental & Clinical Cancer Research. 2020;**39**:213

[111] Williams AB, Li L, Nguyen B, Brown P, Levis M, Small D. Fluvastatin inhibits FLT3 glycosylation in human and murine cells and prolongs survival of mice with FLT3/ITD leukemia. Blood. 2012;**120**:3069-3079

[112] Al-Wahaibi LH, Al-Saleem MSM, Ahmed OAA, Fahmy UA, Alhakamy NA, Eid BG, et al. Optimized conjugation of Fluvastatin to HIV-1 TAT displays enhanced pro-apoptotic activity in HepG2 cells. International Journal of Molecular Sciences. 2020;**21**:4138

[113] Zhang S, Doudican NA, Quay E, Orlow SJ. Fluvastatin enhances sorafenib cytotoxicity in melanoma cells via modulation of AKT and JNK signaling pathways. Anticancer Research. 2011;**31**:3259-3265

[114] Cheng Y, Luo R, Zheng H, Wang B, Liu Y, Liu D, et al. Synergistic anti-tumor efficacy of sorafenib and fluvastatin in hepatocellular carcinoma. Oncotarget. 2017;**8**:23265-23276

[115] Nishiya M, Yasuhira S, Shibazaki M, Oikawa H, Masuda T, Maesawa C. Fluvastatin exerts an antitumor effect in vemurafenib-resistant melanoma cells. Anti-Cancer Drugs. 2019;**30**:451-457

[116] Iizuka-Ohashi M, Watanabe M, Sukeno M, Morita M, Hoang NTH, Kuchimaru T, et al. Blockage of the mevalonate pathway overcomes the apoptotic resistance to MEK inhibitors with suppressing the activation of Akt in cancer cells. Oncotarget. 2018;**9**:19597-19612

[117] Otahal A, Aydemir D, Tomasich E, Minichsdorfer C. Delineation of cell death mechanisms induced by synergistic effects of statins and erlotinib in non-small cell lung cancer cell (NSCLC) lines. Scientific Reports. 2020;**10**:959

[118] Fromigué O, Hamidouche Z, Marie PJ. Statin-induced inhibition of 3-hydroxy-3-methyl glutaryl coenzyme a reductase sensitizes human osteosarcoma cells to anticancer drugs. The Journal of Pharmacology and Experimental Therapeutics. 2008;**325**:595-600

[119] Kitagawa K, Moriya K, Kaji K, Saikawa S, Sato S, Nishimura N, et al. Atorvastatin augments

gemcitabine-mediated anti-cancer effects by inhibiting yes-associated protein in human cholangiocarcinoma cells. International Journal of Molecular Sciences. 2020;**21**:7588

[120] Chen J, Bi H, Hou J, Zhang X, Zhang C, Yue L, et al. Atorvastatin overcomes gefitinib resistance in KRAS mutant human non-small cell lung carcinoma cells. Cell Death & Disease. 2013;**4**:e814

[121] Ghasemi M, Malek M, Javanmard SH, Ghasemi A, Esfahani HN, Vaseghi G. Atorvastatin enhances the apoptotic effects of tamoxifen on melanoma cancer cells. Bratislavské Lekárske Listy. 2019;**120**:752-756

[122] Goda AE, Elsisi AE, Sokkar SS, Abdelrazik NM. Enhanced in vivo targeting of estrogen receptor alpha signaling in murine mammary adenocarcinoma by nilotinib/rosuvastatin novel combination. Toxicology and Applied Pharmacology. 2020;**404**:115185

[123] El Sayed I, Helmy MW, El-Abhar HS. Inhibition of SRC/FAK cue: A novel pathway for the synergistic effect of rosuvastatin on the anti-cancer effect of dasatinib in hepatocellular carcinoma. Life Sciences. 2018;**213**:248-257

[124] Altwairgi AK, Alghareeb WA, AlNajjar FH, Alhussain H, Alsaeed E, Alsharm AA. Atorvastatin in combination with radiotherapy and temozolomide for glioblastoma: A prospective phase II study. Investigational New Drugs. 2021;**39**(1):226-231. DOI: 10.1007/s10637-020-00992-5

[125] Sylvester PW. Synergistic anticancer effects of combined γ-tocotrienol with statin or receptor tyrosine kinase inhibitor treatment. Genes & Nutrition. 2012;**7**(1):63-74. DOI: 10.1007/s12263-011-0225-y

[126] Mao B, Zhang Q, Ma L, Zhao P, Yan P. Overview of research into mTOR inhibitors. Molecules. 2022;**27**(16):5295. DOI: 10.3390/molecules27165295

[127] Nolting S, Maurer J, Spottl G, Aristizabal PET, Reuther C, Young K, et al. Additive anti-tumor effects of lovastatin and Everolimus In vitro through simultaneous inhibition of Signaling pathways. PLoS One. 2015;**10**(12):e0143830

[128] Asari K, Sun WT, Kok ZH, Lam YH, Ng BL, et al. Simvastatin enhances the efficacy of nilotinib in chronic myeloid leukemia by post-translational modification and drug transporter modulation. Anti-Cancer Drugs. 2021;**32**(5):526-536. DOI: 10.1097/CAD.0000000000001028

[129] Lin CK, Liu ST, Chang CC, Huang SM. Regulatory mechanisms of fluvastatin and lovastatin for the p21 induction in human cervical cancer HeLa cells. PLoS One. 2019;**14**:e0214408. DOI: 10.1371/journal.pone.0214408

[130] Mao WJ, Cai Y, Chen D, Jiang G, Xu YR, et al. Statins shapes inflamed tumor microenvironment and enhances immune checkpoint blockade in non-small cell lung cancer. JCI Insight (Metabolism Oncology). 2022;7(18):e161940. DOI: 10.1172/jci.insight.161940

[131] Kansal V, Burnham AJ, Kinney BLC, Saba NF, Paulos C, Lesinki GB, et al. Statins drugs enhance responses to immune checkpoint blockade in head and neck cancer models. Journal for Immunotherapy of Cancer. 2023;**11**(1):e005940. DOI: 10.1136/jitc-2022-005940

[132] Tripathi S, Gupta E, Galande S. Statins as anti-tumor agents: A paradigm for repurposed drugs. Cancer Reports. 2024;7(5):e2078. DOI: 10.1002/cnr2.2078

[133] Karlic H, Thaler R, Gerner C, Grunt T, Proestling K, Haider F, et al. Inhibition of the mevalonate pathway affects epigenetic regulation in cancer cells. Cancer Genetics. 2015;**208**(5):241-252. DOI: 10.1016/j.cancergen.2015.03.008

[134] Xu H, Ye D, Ren M, Zhang Bi F. Ferroptosis in the tumor microenvironment: Perspectives for immunotherapy. Trends in Molecular Medicine. 2021b;**27**(9):856-867. DOI: 10.1016/j.molmed.2021.06.014

[135] Saha S, Lo OK, Duan X, Chen H, Wang Q. Breast tumor initiating cell fate is regulated by microenvironmental cues from an extracellular matrix. Integrative Biology. 2012;**4**:897-904. DOI: 10.1039/c2ib20034a

[136] Karimi JA, Asgari R, Keshavarz SS, Rezael N. Nanomedicine marvels: Crafting the future of cancer therapy with innovative statin nano-formulation strategies. Nanoscale Advances. 2024;**6**(23):5748-5772. DOI: 10.1039/d4na00808a

Chapter 2

Perspective Chapter: Sex Differences during Statin Therapy in Patients with Elevated Risk of Cardiovascular Disease and Cancer

Tatjana Ábel and Éva Csajbókné Csobod

Abstract

The latest guidelines recommend statin therapy for patients with established cardiovascular disease (CVD), type 2 diabetes mellitus (T2DM) or metabolic dysfunction-associated steatotic liver disease (MASLD). Women are often under-represented in clinical trials, which may lead to less reliable data on sex differences in the effects of statin therapy. Few data have been published on possible sex differences in the effect of statin treatment in patients with T2DM or MASLD. The ageing of the world population is contributing to the increasing prevalence of both CVD and malignant diseases. Recently, the potential activity of statins against various types of cancer has also been described. However, few and in some cases conflicting results have been reported on the association between sex differences in statin treatment and cancer risk. The aim of this chapter is to summarise the possible sex differences in the effect of statin treatment on the development of different cancer types and CVD risk factors in patients with T2DM and MASLD.

Keywords: cancer, cardiovascular disease, diabetes, gender, LDL cholesterol, MASLD

1. Introduction

Cardiovascular disease (CVD) remains the leading cause of morbidity and mortality among adults, despite improvements in prevention and treatment [1, 2]. According to the American Heart Association's (AHA) Statistical Report 2024, between 2017 and 2020, men had a higher prevalence of both total CVD (52.4 vs. 44.8%) and coronary heart disease (CHD) (8.7 vs. 5.8%) compared to women [2].

The current practice guidelines state that low-density lipoprotein cholesterol (LDL-C) remains the primary goal of therapy, with the optimal level of LDL-C reduction being tailored to the risk level of each risk group [3, 4]. As an inhibitor of 3-hydroxy-3-methylglutaryl coenzyme A (HMG-CoA) reductase, statin therapy is a cornerstone of CVD risk reduction through its reduction of LDL-C and other pleiotropic effects [5, 6]. These results motivated us to observe possible anti-cancer potentials of statins.

Since the 1990s, most large multicentre primary and secondary prevention statin trials have included women, but the proportion of women participants has been lower than that of men [7–12]. Nevertheless, both primary and secondary prevention studies have shown that there is no significant difference between men and women in the safety and effectiveness of statin treatment in preventing CVD [7–12]. However, fewer results have been published on possible sex differences in statin treatment in people with certain diseases associated with high CVD risk (type 2 diabetes (T2DM), metabolic dysfunction-associated steatotic liver disease (MASLD)). Clinical data are scanty on statin treatment of cancer risks in CVD patients.

Recently, the potential activity of statins against various types of cancer has also been described [13]. Assessing the potential cancer risks associated with the use of statins is crucial to ensure the safety of women and men taking statins long-term.

The aim of this chapter is to summarise the possible sex differences in statin treatment to reduce the risk of developing different types of cancer and CVD risk factors in patients with T2DM and MASLD.

2. Sex differences during statin therapy with high CVD risk patients

2.1 Sex differences during statin therapy in patients with type 2 diabetes

Patients with type 2 diabetes (T2DM) have a higher prevalence and worse prognosis of CHD compared to non-diabetic individuals, perhaps due to poor endothelial injury recovery [14–16].

Researchers from the Framingham Study first time reported that CVD risk differs between men and women with diabetes [17]. Men who had diabetes at baseline or who were diagnosed with diabetes, in the first 16 years of follow-up had double risk of cardiovascular mortality compared with men without diabetes, whereas the risk was 4.5 times higher in women with diabetes than in women without diabetes [17]. A meta-analysis by Peters et al. found that women with T2DM had a more than 40% higher risk of developing CHD than men with diabetes [18]. Recently, a meta-analysis reported that women with diabetes had a 30% higher risk of CVD death, a 58% greater risk of CHD death, 8% higher possibility of stroke death and 13% greater risk of all-cause mortality than diabetic men [19]. There are probably several reasons for the sex differences in CVD risk and events in patients with T2DM, and these are still poorly understood (see **Table 1**) [20–33].

T2DM and dyslipidaemia, which is common in these patients, are considered major CVD risk factors [3, 4]. Several clinical trials have demonstrated significant CHD risk reduction with statin treatment in patients with diabetes, in primary and secondary prevention [4, 34–36]. Current guidelines recommend early and intensive use of statins for lipid control in patients with diabetes [37, 38].

The sex difference is not related to the efficacy of statins, as evidenced from randomised clinical trials. Trials showed that the identical statin treatment results showed same reduction in LDL-C levels in men and women [4]. However, the literature remains contradictory and limited on other possible determinants of sex differences in relation to statins (see **Table 2**) [26, 39–44].

Factors	References
At diagnosis of T2DM, women had higher CV risk factors (BMI, body weight, systolic blood pressure) compared to men.	[19]; [20]
CV risk factors are more prevalent in women with T2DM compared to men with T2DM (obesity, elevated HbA1c and blood pressure, smoking, high triglycerides and LDL-C levels)	[21]; [22]; [23]; [24]; [25]
Sex differences in hormonal pathophysiology (men with T2DM have lower testosterone levels compared to men without T2DM. Women with T2DM have higher testosterone levels than women without T2DM)	[21]; [26]
Race/ethnicity (non-Hispanic, black), socio-economic status (low), healthcare utilisation factors, also associated with sex-related differences in patients with T2DM	[25]; [27]; [28]
Prescription of cardiovascular risk-reducing medicines is lower for women than for men with T2DM (statins, angiotensin-converting enzyme inhibitors, aspirin).	[29]; [30]; [31]; [32]
The use of androgen deprivation therapy (ADT), especially gonadotropin-releasing hormone (GnRH) agonists, in men with prostate cancer (especially in men over 60 years of age) increases the risk of CVD.	[13]
Among the oestrogen receptor modulators in women with breast cancer, tamoxifen therapy increases the risk of venous thromboembolism (VTE). Aromatase inhibitor therapy (letrozole, anastrozole or exemestane) increases the risk of developing CVD.	[13]

BMI = Body Mass Index; CV = cardiovascular; LDL-C = LDL-cholesterol; T2DM = Type 2 diabetes mellitus.

Table 1.
Potential factors associated with sex differences in CVD risk and events in patients with T2DM.

Factors	References
Women are prescribed statins less often than men with T2DM	[38–42]
Women were less likely than men with T2DM to receive statins with a higher potency.	[39]
Statin treatment adherency lower in women than in men with T2DM	[25, 43]
Race, healthcare utilisation factors also associated with sex-related differences in patients with T2DM	[25, 39, 44]

T2DM = Type 2 diabetes mellitus.

Table 2.
Possible factors of statin-related sex differences in CVD risk and events in patients with T2DM.

A recent study found that men with T2DM were more likely prone than women with T2DM to receive statin therapy, regardless of duration of diabetes [42]. Consequently, women were less likely prone than men to achieve the total cholesterol target [42]. Although Stedman et al. recruited patients from only one region of the UK, Salford is recognised as a known diabetes centre [42]. Ambrož et al. studied whether there is a sex difference in the time to start therapy and prescription of statins in patients with T2DM [43]. Their results showed that both the statin initiation (19.7 vs. 24.7%; odds ratio (OR) 0.75; 95% confidence interval (CI) 0.58–0.96) and statin prescription (58.7 vs. 63.9%; OR 0.80, 95% CI 0.73–0.89) were less in females with T2DM than in males. The study investigated T2DM patients including in primary care, therefore these findings are not fully generalisable to T2DM patients treated in other settings.

Vimalananda et al. examined 21,780 women and 646,429 men, aged 50–75 years with diabetes. Their results showed that women were less likely than men to be taking medium or high-dose statins (52 vs. 57%), which may explain why women were less likely to reach their LDL-C target. Although adherence to statin therapy was nearly equal for both sexes, women were less likely than men to visit a community outpatient clinic [40]. In contrast, in the study by Billimek et al. more women reported non-adherence to statins than men with T2DM because of statin's side effects (47.2% vs. 36.8%; $p = 0.024$) [44].

Gamboa et al. studied whether there are race or sex differences in statin use and LDL-C control in patients with T2DM [26]. They concluded that 66% of white men, 57.8% of black men, 55% of white women and 53.6% of black women used statin therapy, respectively, $p < 0.001$ [26]. After adjusting for healthcare utilisation factors, they were shown that LDL-C control among those taking statins was lower among black men, white women as well as black women than white men (prevalence ratios [95% CI]: 0.85 [0.79–0.93], 0.89 [0.82–0.96] and 0.73 [0.67–0.80], respectively, $p < 0.001$) [26].

The study by Russo et al. included a total of 415,294 (45.3% female) patients with T2DM from 236 diabetes centres in Italy [45]. In the outpatient centres, lipid profiles were checked in ~75% of subjects, less often in women than in men, regardless of age, which may be reason related to the fact that women felt less at risk of CVD compared to men [45]. In addition, among patients with T2DM, women were more likely than men to fail to reach the LDL-C target.

2.2 Sex differences during statin therapy in patients with MASLD

Steatotic liver disease (SLD) is a public health concern affecting globally that raises the incidence of CVD [46–48]. Metabolic dysfunction-associated steatotic liver disease (MASLD) is found in 25–45% of the general population and may be present in as high as 70% of patients with T2DM or CVD [49]. MASLD can lead to the development of metabolic-associated steatohepatitis (MASH), a disease characterised by damage and inflammation of hepatocyte and the development of liver fibrosis. The liver fibrosis progression increases the risk of cirrhosis and hepatocellular carcinoma (HCC), both of which are associated with high mortality [50].

Statins can be safely given to individuals with MASLD without increased risk of liver toxicity [51, 52]. This was demonstrated in a recent meta-analysis by Dai et al., which showed that the administration of statins in the management of MASLD and MASH resulted in significantly improving the histological and biochemical biomarkers, especially in patients with hyperlipidaemia [53]. In a study by Ciardullo et al., the effect of statin treatment in patients with T2DM on the risk of liver fibrosis and cirrhosis was examined compared to non-statin-treated patients [54]. The use of statins was linked to a lower risk of both developed liver fibrosis (OR 0.35, 95% CI 0.13–0.90, $p = 0.037$) and cirrhosis (OR 0.09, 95% CI 0.02–0.44, $p = 0.01$). Subgroup analyses showed that this correlation was more pronounced in female patients [54]. In contrast, results from a recent study showed that men may benefit more from statin use in sex-specific analysis, with a significant association between liver-related mortality and HCC (HR, 0.53; 95% CI, 0.30–0.95; $p = 0.03$) [55]. The latest clinical practice guidelines do not discriminate between sexes and recommend statins for the treatment of dyslipidaemic patients with MASLD and MASH with compensated cirrhosis [56].

In MASLD patients, prescribing statins does not appear to be sufficient, as trial results suggest that at least 50% of MASLD patients with an indication and 33% of MASLD patients with CVD are not receiving treatment [57, 58].

Few and conflicting data have been reported on possible differences in statin prescribing and treatment between sexes [59–62]. The study by Thomson et al. involved 2214 patients with MASLD [60]. The mean age of the patients was 62 years, 80.2% were white and 61.1% were women. At baseline, 26.2% had compensated cirrhosis and 20.1% suffered from decompensated cirrhosis. Their results showed that women were less likely to take statins than men, even after adjusting for cardiovascular risk factors and liver disease severity (58.9 vs. 63.8%; $p < 0.019$) [60]. In contrast, Del Ben et al. found that although only 44% of patients with MASLD and an indication for statin therapy were taking statins, a higher proportion of these were women and not men [61]. However, a recent study examining statin prescribing patterns in patients with MASLD ($n = 1238$, 64% women) in primary care showed that there was no significant difference between women and men ($p = 0.818$) [62].

Clinically important hepatotoxicity associated with statin treatment is an extremely rare side effect. In contrast, asymptomatic and usually transient liver transaminase enzyme elevation may be a more common side effect, occurring mainly during the first 12 weeks of statin therapy [62, 63].

Studies to date suggest that the main reason for inappropriate prescription and discontinuation of statins in patients with MASLD/MASH is still the fear of a possible further increase in transaminases and thus the development of liver-related drug damage [62–64]. This may also explain the possible sex differences in the results.

3. Sex differences in the risk of developing cancer during statin treatment

The ageing of the world population is contributing to the increasing prevalence of both CVD and malignant diseases [13]. Still, it is dilemma if statins cause androgen deprivation or increase the prevalence of malignancy (see **Figure 1**) [65]. Recent trend is in favour of statins in combination therapy to prevent one from cancers [66, 67]. The evidence so far suggests that statins may exert their anti-cancer effects through different possible mechanisms (see **Figure 2**) [68–70].

Most of the studies published so far have shown an inverse association between the use of statins and various cancer risks, but some have shown different results [7–71].

Meta-analyses of randomised controlled trials (RCTs) have shown no significant association between statin use and overall cancer incidence [71, 72]. Some observational studies have found a reduced risk of several cancers, such as colorectal, pancreatic, prostate and lung cancers, among people taking statins [73, 74]. Another observational study has found no significant association with colorectal cancer, breast, pancreatic and prostate cancers [75]. In addition, some studies have suggested a possible increased risk of certain malignancies, notably colon, prostate and lung cancers [76, 77]. Marrone et al., examining participants in the Atherosclerosis Risk in Communities Study, found an inverse association of shorter duration of statin use with the incidence of bladder cancer in men (<10 years: HR = 1.67, 95% CI = 1.02–2.73) [73]. Still, the differences of testosterone versus progesterone or oestrogen in statin therapy responses are not confirmed yet.

In cancer patients, the risk of CVD may be increased due to shared risk factors, such as cancer-therapy related cardiovascular (CV) toxicity and pathophysiological mechanisms associated with the underlying malignancy [13]. Cancer-therapy related CV toxicity can be influenced by a number of risk factors, such as age, type of cancer, pre-existing CV risk factors or CVD, type or dose or frequency and duration of current and possibly previous cardiotoxic oncological therapy (13). Advances in the

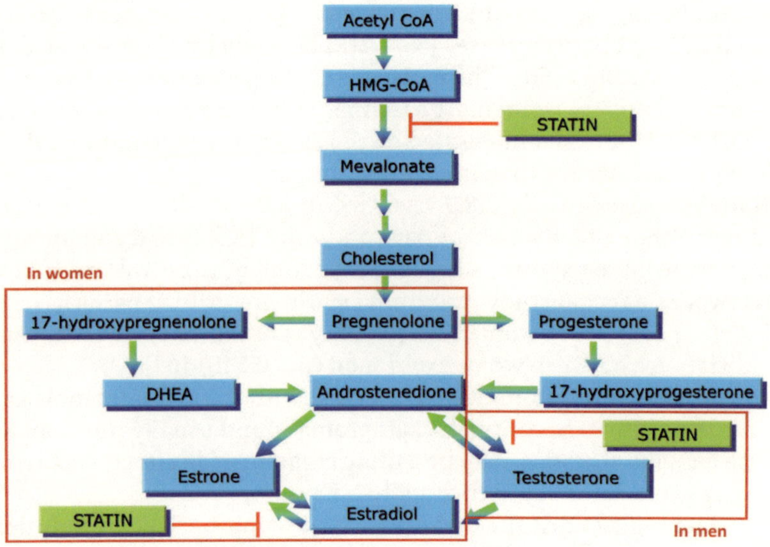

Figure 1.
Cholesterol-lowering and androgen deprivation effects of statins. CoA = co-enzyme A; DHEA = dehydroepiandrosterone; HMG-CoA = 3-hydroxy-3-methylglutaryl coenzyme A.

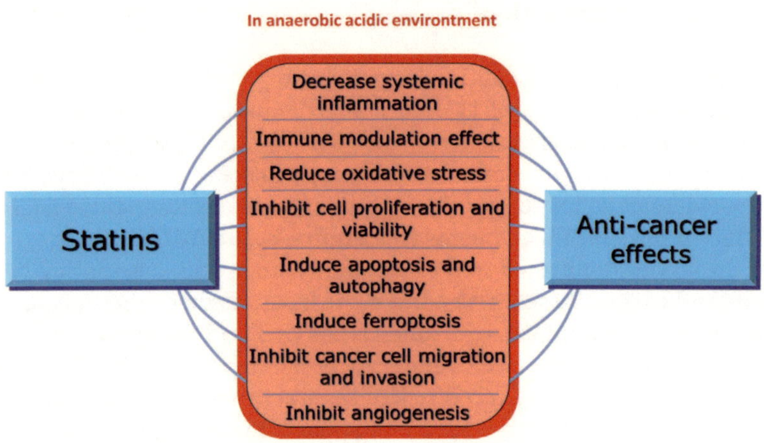

Figure 2.
Possible mechanisms of the anti-cancer effects of statins [68–70].

early diagnosis and management of cancer have resulted in an increased survival rate, an increasing proportion of cancer patients are entering the group at higher risk of CVD [13]. Current cardio-oncology guidelines recommend assessing CV risk before starting cancer chemotherapy and starting statin therapy in combination as early as possible if necessary (see **Table 3**) [13, 78]. According to cardio-oncology guidelines, statins should be considered for primary prevention in adult cancer patients at high and very high risk of CV toxicity (see **Table 4**) [13, 78].

Kobo et al. from the National Health and Nutrition Examination Survey observed both cancer and non-cancer patients taking statins (n = 17.050, 1684 patients had

Drugs
Aromatase inhibitors (anastrozole, letrozole, exemestane)
Asparaginase
Bexarotene
Cyclosporine
Copanlisib
Corticosteroids
Crizotinib
Dasatinib
Duvelisib
Everolimus
Idealisib
Lorlatinib
Mitotane
Nilotinib
Pegaspargase
Ponatinib
Ruxolitinib
Temsirolimus
Tretinoin

Table 3.
Chemotherapies that may increase the risk of developing dyslipidaemia [13, 78].

CV risk group	LDL-C target (mg/dL)
Low risk (SCORE < 1%)	< 116
Moderate risk (SCORE ≥ 1 and < 5%)	< 100
High risk (SCORE ≥ 5 and < 10%)	< 70
Very high risk (SCORE ≥ 10%) (primary or secondary prevention)	< 55
(targets are the same as the latest ESC and AHA recommendations for non-cancer patients [3, 4]).	

Table 4.
LDL-C targets for cancer patients [13, 78].

cancer) [79]. Study results show that among individuals indicated for statin therapy, men were more likely to use statins compared to women, regardless of their cancer status. However, there was more likelihood of both males and females with cancer using statins compared to individuals without cancer, but the difference was more striking for males (75.8 vs. 57.4% and 45.4 vs. 39.6% for men and women, respectively, both $p < 0.001$) [79]. First reason for these results may be that the cancer patients in their study were older, had higher rates of diabetes, hypertension, hyperlipidaemia and established CVD than the patients without cancer. Second reason may be that cancer patients had higher rates of access to health care [79].

3.1 Statin treatment and risk of hepatocellular cancer development

In 2022, liver cancer was the sixth most frequent cancer and the third leading cause of cancer death worldwide [80]. Hepatocellular carcinoma (HCC) represents more than 90% of primary liver cancers. Although hepatitis B and C viral infections (HBV and HCV) are major risk factors for HCC worldwide, the increasing prevalence of obesity, diabetes and MASLD had a greater role in hepatocarcinogenesis [81].

In most geographic regions of the world, HCC incidence and mortality rates are about 2–3 times higher in men than in women [82]. This is mainly due to the fact that men are more likely to have some of the established risk factors for liver cancer, such as HBV and HCV infection, excessive alcohol consumption, smoking and T2DM [83, 84].

The effect of statin treatment on the development of HCC in the general population was investigated [55]. The results showed that the development of HCC was lower primarily in men who were diabetic and had a high Fibrosis-4 index at baseline. This effect of statins was found in favour to be time- and dose-dependent. In women, no benefit was found for statin treatment (see **Table 5**) [55].

Goh et al. observed that HBV-infected patients receiving statin treatment ($n = 713$, 67.6% male) were followed for a median follow-up of 7.2 years for the risk of developing HCC [85]. Their results showed that men had a significantly lower rate of HCC development during statin treatment compared to women according to multivariable Cox regression model with time-dependent covariates (HR, 2.24; 95% CI, 1.86–2.69; $p < 0.001$) [85]. Possiblly, progesterone, oestrogens in females and testosterone in males affect the androgens made from cholesterol differently. These androgens may be deprived by statin-induced mevalonate, squalene, cholesterol-lowering (androgen deprivation therapy, ADT) towards HCC (see **Figure 1**).

However, neither the pathogenesis nor the risk factors that cause the sex differences in the reduction of HCC development during statin treatment are yet known.

3.2 Statin treatment and risk of other cancer development

Colorectal cancer is reported to be the fourth most common cancer in men and the third in women worldwide by 2022 [80]. In their study, Lee et al. examined the risk of colorectal cancer in patients taking statins compared with statin nonusers [86]. Of the 16,588 male participants, 378 (2.3%) developed colorectal cancer during the median follow-up period of 12.7 years, while 239 (1.6%) of the 14,561 female participants developed colorectal cancer. Statin users were classified into high and low users based on medication possession ratio. Among men, those with high statin use had the lowest incidence of total colon, proximal colon and rectal cancers (all $p < 0.05$). Women had also lower incidence of total colon ($p = 0.032$) and rectal cancers ($p = 0.002$) compared to nonusers.

The effect of statin treatment on the risk of developing *renal cell carcinoma* (RCC) has shown conflicting results between the sexes. A recent study found that statin use was not associated with an overall risk of RCC ($n = 661$) [87]. However, in women with high-grade kidney disease in the Nurses' Health Study (NHS) cohort, statin treatment was associated with an increased risk of RCC (HR 1.75, 95% CI 1.07–2.85), and in men who had received statin treatment for 4 years or more, statin treatment was associated with an increased risk of clear cell RCC (HR 1.65, 95% CI 1.10–2.47) [87]. However, this study had a small sample size and a relatively short duration (4+ years), so the authors suggest that further studies are needed to clarify this relationship. In contrast, results from a case-control study showed ($n = 1446$; 91.7% were

Study	Patients	Intervention	Duration	Findings
Vell et al. [55]	1.785.491 individuals (56% men, 49% women)	Statins	• UK Biobank: mean follow-up (standard deviation (SD)): 11.9 (1.9) years; • Penn Medicine BioBank: mean follow-up (SD): 4.7 (2.3) years	In men, statin treatment significantly reduced the risk of developing HCC. (HR, 0.53; 95% CI, 0.30–0.95; p = 0.03). No such association was found in women.
Goh et al. [85]	713 patients infected with HBV and using statins (67.6% men)	Statins	Median follow-up: 7.2 years	Men had significantly lower incidence of HCC compared to women (HR, 2.24; 95% CI, 1.86–2.69; p < 0.001).
Lee et al. [86]	17.737 statin users and 13.412 statin nonusers	Statin treatment compared to nonusers	Median follow-up: 12.7 years	Compared with nonusers, the risk of colorectal cancer is significantly lower in high statin users men (HRs, 95% CIs 0.56 (0.42–0.75) and 0.64 (0.46–0.90)) women.
Michalek et al. [87]	Women from NHS: 100.195 and from NHS II: 91.427; men from HPFS: 45.433	Statins	Women from NHS: 22 years and from NHS II: 16 years; men from HPFS: 26 years	Subgroup analysis: women with high-grade kidney disease increased risk of RCC (HR 1.75, 95% CI 1.07–2.85); and men increased risk of clear cell RCC (HR 1.65, 95% CI 1.10–2.47)
Khurana et al. [88]	483.733 patients (91.7% were men)	Statins	Retrospective nested case–control study	Significantly reduced risk of RCC (48%, adjusted odds ratio 0.52, 95% CI 0.45–0.60)
Cheng et al. [96]	6271 pairs of statin users and nonusers with ESRD	Statins	Follow-up 17 years	The incidence of UTUC was twice as high in women as in men (31.8 vs. 15.9 per 10.000 person-years)

ESRD = End-stage renal disease; HBV = Hepatitis B virus; HCC=Hepatocellular carcinoma; HPFS: Health Professionals Follow-up Study; NHS: Nurses' Health Study; RCC = Renal cell carcinoma; UTUC=Upper tract urothelial carcinoma.

Table 5.
Sex differences in the incidence of various cancers during statin therapy.

men) that statins were significantly protective against the development of RCC (48%, adjusted odds ratio 0.52, 95% confidence interval 0.45–0.60) after controlling for age, sex, smoking and obesity [88].

Statins have an important role in the primary and secondary prevention of cardiovascular events and death in people who have mild-to-moderate chronic kidney disease (CKD) [89, 90]. The KDIGO (Kidney Disease Improving Global Outcome) clinical practice guideline published in 2024 recommended statin monotherapy or statin plus ezetimibe combination therapy for dyslipidaemia in patients with CKD, which still does not clearly recommend statin therapy in advanced CKD or in patients in end-stage renal disease (ESRD) (see **Table 6**) [91]. However, other therapeutic options with different mechanisms of action also reduce the risk of CVD in patients with CKD, such as PCSK9 (proprotein convertase subtilisin/kexin type 9) inhibitors

Recommendations
In adults ≥50 years of age with an estimated glomerular filtration rate (eGFR) < 60 mL/min/1.73 m^2 but not on chronic dialysis or undergoing kidney transplantation, treatment with statin or statin/ezetimibe combination is recommended.
In adults ≥50 years of age with CKD and an eGFR of ≥60 ml/min/1.73 m2, treatment with statin is recommended.
In adults aged 18–49 years with CKD but not treated with chronic dialysis or kidney transplantation who have one or more of the following, statin treatment is recommended: • Known coronary artery disease (myocardial infarction or coronary revascularisation), • diabetes mellitus, • prior ischaemic stroke, or • an estimated 10-year incidence of coronary death or non-fatal myocardial infarction >10%.

Table 6.
The KDIGO guideline recommendations for the management of dyslipidaemia in patients with chronic kidney disease (CKD) [91].

(mainly alirocumab and evolocumab), canakinumab monoclonal antibody targeting interleukin-1β (IL-1β) and colchicine treatment. However, further studies are still needed to confirm these therapies [92–95].

Results from a recent population-based, 17-year follow-up study showed that statin use increased the risk of upper tract urothelial carcinoma (UTUC) in patients with ESRD (n = 6271) (sHR 1.98; 95% CI, 1.28–3.06), but the incidence was twice as high in women than in men (31.8 vs. 15.9 per 10,000 person-years) [96]. This association also held for lipophilic or hydrophilic statin therapy. However, this study had several limitations. In Taiwan, the risk of developing UTUC is increased by an herb used there containing aristolochic acid, and its use in herbal prescriptions was banned in 2003 [96]. However, in this study, the investigators were unable to investigate whether or not exposure to aristolochic acid occurred in the study participants. Furthermore, work history and chemical exposures may have played a role in the risk of UTUC but were not included in the adjustment. The generalisability of the results of the study may also be limited as it was carried out in the framework of the National Health Insurance Database.

In contrast, results of a target trial emulation study showed that statin use had no effect on the incidence of UTUC during the 10-year follow-up period in both sexes, but it should be noted that these patients did not have end-stage renal disease [75].

Despite the fact that statins can affect sex hormone production at different points, the results of the studies summarised have been contradictory (see **Figure 1**) [65, 97]. Although most studies and their cumulative analyses showed that statin treatment was associated with a decrease in total testosterone, this effect was not significant [97, 98]. In patients with prostate cancer receiving ADT, concomitant use of statins has been consistently reported to be beneficial [67, 66]. In a 25-cohort systematic review and meta-analysis by Jayalath et al. involving 119,878 men, statin therapy added to ADT reduced the risk of all-cause mortality by 27% and the risk of prostate cancer-specific mortality by 35% [67]. A similar association was found when comparing 2578 statin users and 2342 nonusers in a study of Asian prostate cancer patients receiving ADT [66]. Over a mean follow-up period of more than 4 years, they found that those who used statins had a significantly lower risk of both prostate cancer-related mortality (weighted hazard ratio [wHR] 0.56 [95% CI 0.48, 0.65], $p < 0.001$) and all-cause mortality (wHR 0.57 [95% CI 0.51, 0.63], $p < 0.001$), irrespective of the type of ADT used [66].

For prostate cancer patients using ADT and breast cancer patients receiving endocrine therapy with no history of CVD, a baseline assessment of CVD risk and 10-year estimates of fatal and non-fatal CVD risk are recommended using the Systematic Coronary Risk Estimation 2 (SCORE2) or the Systematic Coronary Risk Estimation 2-Older Persons (SCORE2-OP) [13]. It is recommended to assess annual CV risk during ADT treatment and in breast cancer patients receiving endocrine therapy with a high 10-year risk of CV events (fatal and non-fatal) [13]. It is recommended to start statin therapy and to achieve LDL-C up to the target level, which is in line with recent European Society of Cardiology (ESC) and AHA recommendations for non-cancer patients (see **Table 4**) [3, 4].

4. Discussion

Reducing LDL-C is an integral part of current guidelines for the management of dyslipidaemia and the prevention and treatment of CVD [3, 4]. Statins are the first-line therapy for the treatment of elevated cholesterol in individuals at increased CV risk, as they are effective in reducing major CVD events and mortality [5, 6].

Women are often under-represented in clinical trials, which can lead to less reliable data on the sex differences in the effects of statin therapy [7, 9]. Several studies suggest that women have poorer control of cardiovascular risk factors, such as obesity, hypertension or hypercholesterolaemia, than their male counterparts [45, 99]. However, it is not clear whether this sex difference is due to progesterone, oestrogen versus testosterone hormonal response, lifestyle- or healthcare utilisation factors, with lower rates of prescribing or taking medication, or higher rates of discontinuation.

To date, a limited number of studies have investigated potential sex differences in long-term statin prescription, adherence, therapy and discontinuation in patients with T2DM. However, the majority of studies have shown that women with T2DM, for a variety of reasons, achieve the LDL-C target at lower rates than men with T2DM [26, 40, 45].

For patients with MASLD, statin therapy is safe and effective, but statins are still under-prescribed in both sexes [57, 58]. However, the reasons for the lower prescription rate are not known, but may be due to fears of further transaminase elevations [62–64].

Disruptions in the mevalonate synthesis pathway caused by statins inhibit cancer growth and lead to apoptotic cell death [96]. Statins also have multiple pleiotropic effects, such as anti-inflammatory properties, suppression of oxidative stress, through which statins may also inhibit carcinogenesis [100–102]. A new statin, pitavastatin, has a favourable pharmacological profile, including a long half-life and minimal metabolism via cytochrome P450 (CYP) enzymes [103]. Studies published so far have shown that pitavastatin, when used in combination with chemotherapy, has anti-cancer activity, e.g. against brain tumours or cervical cancer [104, 105].

The majority of studies published to date have found that statin treatment is dose- and time-dependently inversely correlated with risk of cancer development [55, 85, 86]. Results from several ongoing clinical trials are expected in men and women with cardio-oncological cancer who are receiving combination therapy with statins (see **Table 7**) [106].

Trials
Preventing Anthracycline Cardiovascular Toxicity With Statins (PREVENT). (ClinicalTrials.gov ID NCT01988571)
Statins for the Primary Prevention of Heart Failure in Patients Receiving Anthracycline Pilot Study. (ClinicalTrials.gov ID NCT03186404)
Fish Oil Versus Statins Versus Placebos in Reducing Artial Fibrillation in Patients Undergoing Thoracic Surgery for Lung Cancer. (ClinicalTrials.gov ID NCT01259284)
Atorvastatin Treatment of Cavernous Angiomas with Symptomatic Haemorrhage Exploratory Proof of Concept (AT CASH EPOC) Trial. (ClinicalTrials.gov ID NCT02603328)
Statins and prOgression of Coronary atheRosclerosis in melanomA Patients Treated with chEckpoint inhibitorS. (ClinicalTrials.gov ID NCT05180942)
Detection and Prevention of Anthracycline-Related Cardiac Toxicity with Concurrent Simvastatin. (ClinicalTrials.gov ID NCT02096588)
Donor Atorvastatin Treatment in Preventing Severe Acute GVHD After Nonmyeloablative Peripheral Blood Stem Cell Transplant in Patients With Haematological Malignancies. (ClinicalTrials.gov ID NCT01527045)
Rosuvastatin in Treating Women With Cardiovascular Complications Who Are Undergoing Chemotherapy For Breast Cancer. (ClinicalTrials.gov ID NCT01051401)

Table 7.
Ongoing clinical trials of combination therapy with statins in men and women with cardio-oncological cancer [106].

5. Conclusion

The statin therapy should be encouraged in both sexes for patients with T2DM and MASLD, as it improves lipid profile and reduces CV risk. Statin treatment in combination with chemotherapy is safe to continue in the long term for both men and women, given the risk of developing various cancers such as cardio-oncologic diseases and HCC. However, the reasons for possible sex differences in statin ADT treatment are not yet known and further research is needed to understand these so that ADT statin treatment strategies can be optimised accordingly if necessary.

Funding

None.

Conflict of interest

The authors declare no conflict of interest.

DOI: http://dx.doi.org/10.5772/intechopen.1010879

Author details

Tatjana Ábel* and Éva Csajbókné Csobod
Department of Dietetics and Nutritional Sciences, Faculty of Health Sciences, Semmelweis University, Budapest, Hungary

*Address all correspondence to: abelt@t-online.hu

References

[1] World Health Organization. The Top 10 Causes of Death. 2024. Available from: https://www.who.int/news-room/fact-sheets/detail/the-top-10-causes-of-death

[2] Martin SS, Aday AW, Almarzooq ZI, et al. 2024 heart disease and stroke statistics: A report of US and global data from the American Heart Association. Circulation. 2024;**149**:e347-e913

[3] Byrne RA, Rossello X, Coughlan JJ, et al. 2023 ESC guidelines for the management of acute coronary syndromes. European Heart Journal. 2023;**44**:3720-3826

[4] Grundy SM, Stone NJ, Bailey AL. AHA/ACC/AACVPR/AAPA/ABC/ACPM/ADA/AGS/APhA/ASPC/NLA/PCNA guideline on the Management of Blood Cholesterol: Executive summary: A report of the American College of Cardiology/American Heart Association task force on clinical practice guidelines. Journal of the American College of Cardiology. 2019;**73**:3168-3209

[5] Collins R, Reith C, Emberson J, et al. Interpretation of the evidence for the efficacy and safety of statin therapy. Lancet. 2016;**388**:2532-2561

[6] Oesterle A, Laufs U, Liao JK. Pleiotropic effects of statins on the cardiovascular system. Circulation Research. 2017;**120**:229-243

[7] Downs JR, Clearfield M, Weis S, et al. Primary prevention of acute coronary events with lovastatin in men and women with average cholesterol levels: Results of AFCAPS/TexCAPS. Air force/Texas coronary atherosclerosis prevention study. Journal of the American Medical Association. 1998;**279**:1615-1622

[8] Ridker PM, Danielson E, Fonseca FA, et al. Rosuvastatin to prevent vascular events in men and women with elevated C-reactive protein. The New England Journal of Medicine. 2008;**359**:2195-2207

[9] Scandinavian Simvastatin Survival Study Group. Randomised trial of cholesterol lowering. In 4444 patients with coronary heart disease: The Scandinavian simvastatin survival study (4S). Lancet. 1994;**344**:1383-1389

[10] Schwartz GG, Olsson AG, Ezekowitz MD, et al. Effects of atorvastatin on early recurrent ischemic events in acute coronary syndromes: The MIRACL study: A randomized controlled trial. Journal of the American Medical Association. 2001;**285**:1711-1718

[11] Cannon CP, Braunwald E, McCabe CH, et al. Intensive versus moderate lipid lowering with statins after acute coronary syndromes. The New England Journal of Medicine. 2004;**350**:1495-1504

[12] LaRosa JC, Grundy SM, Waters DD, et al. Intensive lipid lowering with atorvastatin in patients with stable coronary disease. The New England Journal of Medicine. 2005;**352**:1425-1435

[13] Lyon AR, López-Fernández T, Couch LS, et al. 2022 ESC guidelines on cardio-oncology developed in collaboration with the European Hematology Association (EHA), the European Society for Therapeutic Radiology and Oncology (ESTRO) and the international cardio-oncology society (IC-OS): Developed by the task force on cardio-oncology of the European Society of Cardiology (ESC). European Heart Journal. 2022;**43**:4229-4361

[14] Kannel WB. Lipids, diabetes and coronary heart disease: Insights from the Framingham study. American Heart Journal. 1985;**110**:1100-1107

[15] Chatterjee S, Khunti K, Davies MJ. Type 2 diabetes. Lancet. 2017;**389**:2239-2251

[16] Haffner SM, Lehto S, Rönnemaa T, et al. Mortality from coronary heart disease in subjects with type 2 diabetes and in nondiabetic subjects with and without prior myocardial infarction. The New England Journal of Medicine. 1998;**339**:229-234

[17] Garcia MJ, McNamara PM, Gordon T, Kannel WB. Morbidity and mortality in diabetics in the Framingham population. Sixteen Year Follow-Up Study. Diabetes. 1974;**23**:105-111

[18] Peters SAE, Huxley RR, Woodward M. Diabetes as risk factor for incident coronary heart disease in women compared with men: A systematic review and meta-analysis of 64 cohorts including 858.507 individuals and 28.203 coronary events. Diabetologia. 2014;**57**:1542-1551

[19] Wang Y, O'Neil A, Jiao Y, Wang L, Huang J, Lan Y, et al. Sex differences in the association between diabetes and risk of cardiovascular disease, cancer, and all-cause and cause specific mortality: A systematic review and meta-analysis of 5,162,654 participants. BMC Medicine. 2019;**17**:136

[20] Wright AK, Welsh P, Gill JMR, et al. Age-sex-, and ethnicity-related differences in body weight, blood pressure, HbA1c, and lipid levels at the diagnosis of type 2 diabetes relative to people without diabetes. Diabetologia. 2020;**63**:1542-1553

[21] Johnson ML, Preston JD, Rashid CS, et al. Sex differences in type 2 diabetes: An opportunity for personalized medicine. Biology of Sex Differences. 2023;**14**:88

[22] Lyon A, Jackson EA, Kalyani RR, et al. Sex-specific differential in risk of diabetes-related macrovascular outcomes. Current Diabetes Reports. 2015;**15**:85

[23] Ohkuma T, Iwase M, Fujii H, et al. Sex differences in cardiovascular risk, lifestyle, and psychological factors in patients with type 2 diabetes: The Fukuoka diabetes registry. Biology of Sex Differences. 2023;**14**:32

[24] de Ritter R, de Jong M, Vos RC, et al. Sex differences in the risk of vascular disease associated with diabetes. Biology of Sex Differences. 2020;**11**:1

[25] Criqui M, Barrett-Connor E, Holdbrook MJ, et al. Clustering of cardiovascular disease risk factors. Preventive Medicine. 1980;**9**:525-533

[26] Gamboa CM, Colantonio LD, Brown TM, et al. Race-differences in statin use and low-density lipoprotein cholesterol control among people with diabetes mellitus in the reasons for geographic and racial differences in stroke study. Journal of the American Heart Association. 2017;**6**:e004264

[27] Corona G, Monami M, Rastrelli G, et al. Type 2 diabetes mellitus and testosterone: A meta-analysis study. International Journal of Andrology. 2011;**34**:528-540

[28] Weeda ER, Bishu KG, Ward R, et al. Joint effect of race/ethnicity or location of residence and sex on low density lipoprotein-cholesterol among veterans with type 2 diabetes: A 10-year retrospective cohort study. BMC Cardiovascular Disorders. 2020;**20**:449

[29] Collier A, Ghosh S, Hair M, et al. Impact of socioeconomic status and gender on glycaemic control, cardiovascular risk factors and diabetes complications in type 1 and 2 diabetes: A population based analysis from Scottish region. Diabetes and Metabolism. 2015;**41**:145-151

[30] Al-Salameh A, Bouzegaoui NE, Saraval-Gross M. Diabetes and cardiovascular risk according to sex: An overview of epidemiological data from the early Framingham reports to the cardiovascular outcomes trials. Annales d'endocrinologie. 2023;**84**:57-68

[31] Al-Salameh A, Chanson P, Bucher S, et al. Cardiovascular disease in type 2 diabetes: A review of sex-related differences in predisposition and prevention. Mayo Clinic Proceedings. 2019;**94**:287-308

[32] Ferrannini G, De Bacquer D, Vynckier P, et al. Gender differences in screening for glucose perturbations, cardiovascular risk factor management and prognosis in patients with dysglycaemia and coronary artery disease: Results from the ESC-EORP EUROASPIRE surveys. Cardiovascular Diabetology. 2021;**20**:38

[33] Cull CA, Neil HA, Holman RR. Changing aspirin use in patients with type 2 diabetes in the UKPDS. Diabetic Medicine. 2004;**21**:1368-1371

[34] Naci H, Brugts J, Ades T. Comparative tolerability and harms of individual statins: A study-level network meta-analysis of 246,955 participants from 135 randomized, controlled trials. Circulation. Cardiovascular Quality and Outcomes. 2013;**6**:390-399

[35] Taylor F, Huffman MD, Macedo AF, et al. Statins for the primary prevention of cardiovascular disease. Cochrane Database of Systematic Reviews. 2013;**1**:CD004816

[36] Cholesterol Treatment Trialists' (CTT) Collaborators, Kearney PM, Blackwell L, et al. Efficacy of cholesterol-lowering therapy in 18,686 people with diabetes in 14 randomised trials of statins: A meta-analysis. Lancet. 2008;**371**:117-125

[37] American Diabetes Association Professional Practice Committee. Cardiovascular diasease and risk management: Standards of Care in Diabetes – 2024. Diabetes Care. 2024;**47**(Suppl. 1):S179-S218

[38] Cosentino F, Grant PJ, Aboyans V, et al. 2019 ESC guidelines on diabetes, pre-diabetes, and cardiovascular diseases developed in collaboration with the EASD. European Heart Journal. 2020;**41**:255-323

[39] Baviera M, Santalucia P, Coretesi L, Morzona I, Tettamanti M, Avanzini F, et al. Sex differences in cardiovascular outcomes, pharmacologic treatments and indicators of care in patients with newly diagnosed diabetes: Analyses on administrative database. European Journal of Internal Medicine. 2014;**25**:270-275

[40] Vimalananda VG, Miller DR, Hofer TP, et al. Accounting for clinical action reduces estimates of gender disparities in lipid management for diabetic veterans. Journal of General Internal Medicine. 2013;**28**(Suppl. 2):529-535

[41] Huxley R, Barzi F, Woodward M. Excess risk of fatal coronary heart disease associated with diabetes in men and women: Meta-analysis of 37 prospective cohort studies. BMJ. 2006;**332**:73-78

[42] Stedman M, Whyte MB, Laing I, Fryer AA, Torres BM, Robinson A,

et al. Failure to control conventional cardiovascular risk factors in women with type 2 diabetes might explain worse mortality. Diabetes/Metabolism Research and Reviews. 2023;**39**:e3695

[43] Ambrož M, Geelink M, Smits KPJ, de Vries ST, Denig P. Sex disparities in medication prescribing amongst patients with type 2 diabetes mellitus managed in primary care. Diabetic Medicine. 2023;**40**:e14987

[44] Billimek J, Malik S, Sorkin DH, et al. Understanding disparities in lipid management among patients with type 2 diabetes: Gender differences in medication nonadherence after treatment intensification. Women's Health Issues. 2015;**25**:6-12

[45] Russo G, Pintaudi B, Giorda C, et al. Age- and gender-related differences in LDL-cholesterol Management in Outpatients with type 2 diabetes mellitus. International Journal of Endocrinology. 2015;**2015**:957105

[46] Tamaki N, Kimura T, Wakabayashi SI, et al. Long-term clinical outcomes in steatotic liver disease and incidence of liver-related events, cardiovascular events and all-cause mortality. Alimentary Pharmacology and Therapeutics. 2024;**60**:61-69

[47] Kim KS, Hong S, Han K, et al. Association of non-alcoholic fatty liver disease with cardiovascular disease and all cause death in patients with type 2 diabetes mellitus: Nationwide population based study. BMJ. 2024;**384**:e076388

[48] Zannad F, Sanyal AJ, Butler J, Ferreira JP, Girerd N, Miller V, et al. MASLD and MASH at the crossroads of hepatology trials and cardiorenal metabolic trials. Journal of Internal Medicine. 2024;**296**:24-38

[49] Kasper P, Martin A, Lang S, et al. NAFLD and cardiovascular diseases: A clinical review. Clinical Research in Cardiology. 2021;**110**:921-937

[50] Targher G, Corey KE, Byrne CD, Roden M. The complex link between NAFLD and type 2 diabetes mellitus – Mechanisms and treatments. Nature Reviews. Gastroenterology and Hepatology. 2021;**18**:599-612

[51] Athyros VG, Tziomalos K, Gossios TD, Griva T, Anagnostis P, Kargiotis K, et al. Safety and efficacy of long-term statin treatment for cardiovascular events in patients with coronary heart disease and abnormal liver tests in the Greek atorvastatin and coronary heart disease evaluation (GREACE) study: A post-hoc analysis. Lancet. 2010;**376**:1916-1922

[52] Portillo BF, Sanchez P, Lomonaco R, et al. Liver safety of statins in prediabetes or T2DM and nonalcoholic steatohepatitis: Post hoc analysis of a randomized trial. The Journal of Clinical Endocrinology and Metabolism. 2017;**102**:2950-2961

[53] Dai W, Xu B, Li P, Weng J. Statins for the treatment of nonalcoholic fatty liver disease and nonalcoholic steatohepatitis: A systematic review and meta-analysis. American Journal of Therapeutics. 2023;**30**:e17-e25

[54] Ciardullo S, Perseghin G. Statin use is associated with lower prevalence of advanced liver fibrosis in patients with type 2 diabetes. Metabolism. 2021;**121**:154752

[55] Vell MS, Loomba R, Krishnan A, et al. Association of statin use with risk of liver disease, hepatocellular carcinoma and liver-related mortality. JAMA Network Open. 2023;**6**:e2320222

[56] European Association for the Study of the Liver; European Association for the Study of Diabetes; European Association for the Study of Obesity. EASL–EASD–EASO Clinical Practice Guidelines on the management of metabolic dysfunction-associated steatotic liver disease (MASLD): Executive Summary. Diabetologia. 2024;**67**:2375-2392. DOI: 10.1007/s00125-024-06196-3

[57] Thomson MJ, Serper M, Khungar V, Weiss LM, Trinh H, Firpi-Morell R, et al. Prevalence and factors associated with statin use among patients with nonalcoholic fatty liver disease in the TARGET-NASH study. Clinical Gastroenterology and Hepatology. 2022;**20**:458-60.e4

[58] Shahab O, Biswas R, Paik J, Bush H, Golabi P, Younossi ZM. Among patients with NAFLD, treatment of dyslipidemia does not reduce cardiovascular mortality. Hepatology Communications. 2018;**2**:1227-1234

[59] Ábel T, Benczur B, Csobod ÉCS. Sex differences in pathogenesis and treatment of dyslipidemia in patients with type 2 diabetes and steatotic liver disease. Frontiers in Medicine. 2024;**11**:1458025

[60] Thomson MJ, Serper M, Khungar V, et al. Prevalence and factors associated with statin use among with non-alcoholic fatty liver disease in TARGET-NASH. Clinical Gastroenterology and Hepatology. 2022;**20**:458-460

[61] Del Ben M, Baratta F, Polimeni L, et al. Under-prescription of statins in patients with non-alcoholic fatty liver disease. Nutrition, Metabolism, and Cardiovascular Diseases. 2017;**27**:161-167

[62] Schneider AD, Zhang J, Petz CA, et al. Statin prescriptions and progression of advanced fibrosis risk in primary care patients with MASLD. BMJ Open Gastroenterology. 2024;**11**:e001404

[63] Bernhard J, Lukas Galli L, Walter S, Speidl WS, et al. Cardiovascular risk reduction in metabolic dysfunction-associated Steatotic liver disease and metabolic dysfunction-associated steatohepatitis. Current Cardiology Reports. 2025;**27**:28

[64] Calderon RM, Cubeddu LX, Goldberg RB, et al. Statins in the treatment of dyslipidemia in the presence of elevated liver aminotransferase levels: A therapeutic dilemma. Mayo Clinic Proceedings. 2010;**85**:349-356

[65] Glina FPA, Lopes L, R S e S, et al. Do statins decrease testosterone in men? Systemic review and meta-analysis. International Brazilian Journal of Urology. 2024;**18**(50):119-135

[66] Lee YHA, Chan JSK, Hui JMH, et al. Statin use and mortality risk in Asian patients with prostate cancer receiving androgen deprivation therapy: A population-based cohort study. Cancer Medicine. 2024;**13**:e6826

[67] Jayalath VH, Clark R, Lajkosz K, et al. Statin use and survival among men receiving androgen-ablative therapies for advanced prostate cancer. A systematic review and meta-analysis. JAMA Network Open. 2022;**5**:e2242676

[68] Jiang W, Hu JW, He XR, et al. Statins: A repurposed drug to fight cancer. Journal of Experimental and Clinical Cancer Research. 2021;**40**:241

[69] Tripathi S, Gupta E, Galande S. Statins as anti-tumor agents: A paradigm for repurposed drugs. Cancer Reports. 2024;**7**:e2078

[70] Pasha R, Bashir B, Omed D, et al. Impact of lipid-lowering therapy on cancer risk: A narrative review. Clinical Therapeutics. 2024;**46**:411-419

[71] Emberson JR, Kearney PM, Blackwell L, et al. Lack of effect of lowering LDL cholesterol on cancer: Meta-analysis of individual data from 175.000 people in 27 randomised trials of statin therapy. PLoS One. 2012;7:e29849

[72] Bonovas S. Statins: Do they have a potential role in cancer prevention and modifying cancer-related outcomes? Drugs. 2014;**74**:1841-1848

[73] Marrone MT, Mondul AM, Prizment AE, et al. Lipid-lowering drug use and cancer incidence and mortality in the ARIC study. JNCI Cancer Spectrum. 2021;**5**:pkab080

[74] Poynter JN, Gruber SB, Higgins PD, et al. Statins and the risk of colorectal cancer. The New England Journal of Medicine. 2005;**352**:2184-2192

[75] Xu W, Chan L, Danaei G, et al. Long-term statin use and risk of cancers: A target trial emulation study. Journal of Clinical Epidemiology. 2024;**172**:111425

[76] Chang CC, Ho SC, Chiu HF, et al. Statins increase the risk of prostate cancer: A population-based case-control study. The Prostate. 2011;**71**:1818-1824

[77] Vinogradova Y, Coupland C, Hippisley-Cox J. Exposure to statins and risk of common cancers: A series of nested case-control studies. BMC Cancer. 2011;**11**:409

[78] García AM, Mitroi C, Ramos PM, et al. Stratification and management of cardiovascular risk in cancer patients. A consensus document of the SEC, FEC, SEOM, SEOR, SEHH, SEMG, AEEMT, AEEC and AECC. Revista Española de Cardiología (English Edition). 2021;**74**:438-448

[79] Kobo O, Michos ED, Roguin A, et al. Recommended and observed statin use among US adults with and without cancer. European Journal of Preventive Cardiology. 2024;**31**:1251-1257

[80] International Agency for Research on Cancer. World Health Organization. Global Cancer Observatory. Liver. 2022. Available from: https://gco.iarc.who.int/media/globocan/factsheets/cancers/11-liver-and-intrahepatic-bile-ducts-fact-sheet.pdf

[81] Rumgay H, C FJ d M, et al. Global, regional and national burden of primary liver cancer by subtype. European Journal of Cancer. 2022;**161**:108-118

[82] Mc Glynn KA, Petrick JL, El-Serag HB. Epidemiology of hepatocellular carcinoma. Hepatology. 2021;**73**:4-13

[83] Jackson SS, Marks MA, Katki HA, et al. Sex disparities in the incidence of 21 cancer types: Quantification of the contribution of risk factors. Cancer. 2022;**128**:3531-3540

[84] Baecker A, Liu X, La Vecchia C, et al. Worldwide incidence of hepatocellular carcinoma cases attributable to major risk factors. European Journal of Cancer Prevention. 2018;**27**:205-212

[85] Goh MJ, Sinn DH, Kim S, et al. Statin use and the risk of hepatocellular carcinoma in patients with chronic hepatitis B. Hepatology. 2020;**71**:2023-2032

[86] Lee JW, You NY, Kim Y, et al. Statin use and site-specific risk of colorectal cancer in individuals with hypercholesterolemia from the National Health Insurance Service-National

Health Screening Cohort (NHIS-HEALS). Nutrition, Metabolism, and Cardiovascular Diseases. 2019;**29**:701-709

[87] Michalek IM, Graff RE, Sanchez A, et al. Evaluation of statin use and renal cell carcinoma risk identifies sex-specific associations with RCC subtypes. Acta Oncologica. 2023;**62**:988-993

[88] Khurana V, Caldito G, Ankem M. Statins might reduce risk of renal cell carcinoma in humans: Case-control study of 500,000 veterans. Urology. 2008;**71**:118-122

[89] Mathew RO, Rosenson RS, Lyubarova R, Chaudhry R, Costa SP, Bangalore S, et al. Concepts and controversies: Lipid management in patients with chronic kidney disease. Cardiovascular Drugs Ther. 2021;**35**:479-489

[90] Wang H, Naghavi M, Allen C, Barber RM, Bhutta Z, Carter AR, et al. Global, regional, and national life expectancy, all-cause mortality, and cause-specific mortality for 249 causes of death, 1980-2015: A systematic analysis for the global burden of disease study 2015. Lancet. 2016;**388**:1459-1544

[91] KDIGO. Clinical practice guideline for the evaluation and Management of Chronic Kidney Disease. Kidney International. 2024;**2024**(105):S117-S314

[92] Toth PP, Dwyer JP, Cannon CP, et al. Efficacy and safety of lipid lowering by alirocumab in chronic kidney disease. Kidney International. 2018;**93**:1397-1408

[93] Charytan DM, Sabatine MS, Pedersen TR, Im K, Park JG, Pineda AL, et al. Efficacy and safety of evolocumab in chronic kidney disease in the FOURIER trial. Journal of the American College of Cardiology. 2019;**73**:2961-2970

[94] Ridker PM, MacFadyen JG, Everett RM, et al. Inhibition of interleukin-1β by canakinumab and cardiovascular outcomes in patients with chronic kidney disease. Journal of the American College of Cardiology. 2018;**71**:2405-2414

[95] Tardif JC, Kouz S, Waters DD, et al. Efficacy and safety of low-dose colchicine after myocardial infarction. The New England Journal of Medicine. 2019;**381**:2497-2505

[96] Cheng YC, Sung FC, Muo CH, et al. Statin therapy and upper tract urothelial carcinoma risk in hyperlipidemic patients with chronic kidney disease and end-stage kidney disease, a population-based 17-year follow-up study. Renal Failure. 2024;**46**:2402508

[97] Stamerra CA, Di Giosia P, Ferri C, et al. Statin therapy and sex hormones. European Journal of Pharmacology. 2021;**890**:173745

[98] Oluleye OW, Kronmal RA, Folsom AR, et al. Association between statin use and sex hormone in the multi-ethnic study of atherosclerosis cohort. Endocrinology and Metabolism. 2019;**104**:4600-4606

[99] De Smedt D, De Bacquer D, De Sutter J, et al. The gender gap in risk factor control: Effects of age and education on the control of cardiovascular risk factors in male and female coronary patients. The EUROASPIRE IV study by the European Society of Cardiology. International Journal of Cardiology. 2016;**209**:284-290

[100] Konstantinopoulos PA, Karamouzis MV, Papavassiliou AG. Post-translational modifications and regulation of the RAS superfamily of GTPases as anticancer targets. Nature Reviews Drug Discovery. 2007;**6**:541-555

[101] Hippisley-Cox J, Coupland C. Unintended effects of statins in men and women in England and Wales: Population based cohort study using the QResearch database. BMJ. 2010;**340**:c2197

[102] Katz MS. Therapy insight: Potential of statins for cancer chemoprevention and therapy. Nature Clinical Practice. Oncology. 2005;**2**:82-89

[103] Duggan ST. Pitavastatin: A review of its use in the management of hypercholesterolaemia or mixed dyslipidaemia. Drugs. 2012;**72**:565-584

[104] Basso J, Matos AM, Ghavami S, et al. Are we better together? Addressing a combined treatment of pitavastatin and temozolomide for brain cancer. European Journal of Pharmacology. 2024;**985**:177087

[105] Chen YH, Wu JX, Yang SF, et al. Molecular mechanisms underlying the anticancer properties of pitavastatin against cervical cancer cells. International Journal of Molecular Sciences. 2024;**25**:7915

[106] National Library of Medicine. ClinicalTrials.gov. Available from: https://clinicaltrials.gov

Section 2

Nanotechnology and Cardio-Oncology

Chapter 3

Statin Nanoformulation Methods in Cancer Theranosis: Trimodal Therapy

Rakesh Sharma

Abstract

Lipid-lowering statin medications with repurposed anticancer properties have tremendous potentials in cancer treatment and management. Several preclinical evidences have indicated statin's tumor pro-apoptosis and inhibitory functions to arrest angiogenesis, or resistance to metastasis and other critical processes in cancer development. Clinical applications of statin use in oncology suffer from low solubility and bioavailability of statins given with chemodrugs. These challenges are overcome by use of statin–chemodrug nanoformulations as nanomedicines to enhance the statins and chemodrug delivery, solubility, stability, and targeting ability for maximum anticancer therapeutic efficacy with maximum accumulation of nanomedicines in tumors without any side effects. Different statins exert anticancer effects by the specific mechanisms of mevalonate, immune response modulation, and induced apoptosis pathways. The authors propose "trimodal therapy" in the present chapter on development of statin-loaded nanoformulations of liposomes, micelles, and polymeric beads filled with chemo-radiotherapy drugs and with immunotherapy and targeted therapy drugs as hybrid nanomedicines or trimodal therapy, as well as their nanodelivery applications and anticancer properties in tumors to improve cancer treatment and offer better patient outcomes. In conclusion, multiple hybrid nanodrugs, or controlled delivery of statins with other two or more anticancer drugs, enhances the anticancer effects and simultaneously reduces the cardiotoxicity, cytotoxicity, drug resistance, and tumor recurrence to enhance the overall clinical and patient outcomes.

Keywords: nanoformulations, statins, nanomedicines, cancer theranosis, enhanced patient outcome

1. Introduction

Cancer is a state of abnormally high cell division and uncontrolled proliferation and tumor growth without any control on growing, in the forms of recurrent malignant sarcoma, fibroma, metastases, and resistance to drugs. Over 20 million new cancer cases and around 10 million deaths were reported globally in the year 2022 [1]. In the United States alone, 1.9 million new cases with 0.6 million deaths were reported in the year 2023. Cancer is a multifactorial disease due to environment and lifestyle risks. Unfortunately, cancer treatments are invasive with noticeable toxicity; therefore, preventive risk factors and lifestyle modification measures seem very effective.

Statin drugs are established for their anti-antherosclerotic effects with anticancer potential. Basically, statins inhibit the 3-hydroxy-3-methyl-glutaryl-CoA reductase (HMG CoA-R) enzyme to prevent cholesterol synthesis. During cholesterol synthesis, statins may alter the intermediate farnesyl-PP metabolic step in pathway toward autophagy, apoptosis, redox, cell cycle, and immune control steps. Statin-loaded nanomedicine formulation designs are ongoing efforts to treat the cancers as adjunct therapies with chemo-radiotherapy. Other possibilities are statin-loaded nanoformulation methods along with radiation therapy, hyperthermia, immunotherapy, stem cell transplant, and targeted therapy. However, every therapeutic modality has challenges and limitations due to limited efficacy, side effects, or invasiveness. For example, statins show poor solubility, stability and bioavailability. Use of nanostatin chemodrugs caged in liposomes, micelles, chitosan, polymer nanomaterials, and other hybrid delivery systems allows transport of the statins and drugs safely in blood to enhance the statin solubility, stability, and bioavailability with improved drug therapeutic efficacy and low systemic side effects. Recently, targeted therapy by nano-assemblies caging the chemo-radiotherapy medicines has emerged as a precise treatment with high efficacy and least side-effects.

The trimodal therapy is an approach of safe delivery of statins given in combination of chemotherapy and radiotherapy with possible immunotherapy and targeted therapy used in cancer treatment.

The present chapter highlights the use of safe, stable, pH dependent, controlled release drug delivery nanoformulations for statin chemo-radiotherapy drugs used in cancer treatment. Nanotechnology offers the promising methods of design and preparation of drug delivery nanoformulations, modern vaccines, diagnostics, and so forth in cancer treatment. Nanodrug delivery platforms are made of polymeric, lipophilic, or hydrophilic micelles and metallic materials to transport nanomedicines at specific physiological pH conditions with minimal or no toxicity. Chemotherapy is also less invasive with limited side effects and toxicity. Radiation therapy and immunotherapies are more cytotoxic and need attention for their safe nanodelivery, while statins in combination may reduce overall cardiotoxicity due to radiation therapy or immunotherapies.

2. Statins

Statins are made of a polyketide ring structure with a hydroxyl-hexahydro naphthalene ring system attached at C8 and C6 positions on the ring. Statins are classified based on their chemical structure and their solubility properties. Atorvastatin and fluvastatin are synthesized from mevalonate and pyridine. The lovastatin is derived from *Aspergillus terreus* or *Monascus ruber*. The pravastatin is derived from the mevastatin product from *Penicillium citrinum*. Simvastatin is a semi-synthetic statin derived from lovastatin (C8 chemical modified chain). These statins show different solubility profiles. For example, hydrophilic statins (pravastatin and rosuvastatin) easily cross the membrane to reach their target. The lipophilic (simvastatin and atorvastatin) statins stay longer in the bloodstream.

2.1 Concept of statin anticancer functions and nanomedicine

Nanomedicine is defined as "unrestricted entry with anticancer function of nanomaterial carriers filled with statins and/or chemoradiotherapy" drugs (anthracyclins, cyclophosphamide) as safe nanobags or nanospheres of 1×10^{-9} m size, traveling or circulating in the bloodstream or accumulated inside tumor cell organelles without barriers of pH, physiology, or biochemical and mechanical effects. These characteristics make statin-loaded nanoparticles or nanomedicines to be stable, bioavailable, and biocompatible in the tumor microenvironment to use statins as anticancer medicines. Nanocarriers are mainly liposomes, micelles, chitosan, graphene, fullerene, polyethylglycol (PeG), poly-glycolactate (PGLA) polymers, and Qdots. These nanoformulations perform pH-dependent controlled drug release by group transformations. Nanoformulation offers protective action against abnormal tumor enzymes and facilitates the nanomaterial cage opening in tumor blood at the target site.

In the cancer growth suppression or anticancer action, statins modify the mevalonate pathway and down-regulate the proteins of pro-angiogenesis, pro-apoptosis, and endothelial-Akt-derive dnitric oxide at three cross-points to perform endothelial cell proliferation, immunomodulation, and blocking the intracellular adhesion molecules for extracellular adhesion. Statins behave differently at low doses and high doses as anticancer medicines, and they enhance the anticancer efficiency of combination chemo-radiotherapy drugs.

At low dose, statins inhibit the mevalonate pathway by the HMG-CoA reductase enzyme as a defensive lipid-lowering effect (Hippo pathway) against any cross-talk effect of angiogenesis-stimulated migration, endothelium differentiation, uncontrolled cell proliferation, apoptosis, and pleiotropic effects in cardiovascular disease, stroke, thromboembolism, renal disease, rheumatoid arthritis, dementia, fatty liver, diabetes, and neurological disease [2, 3].

At high dose, statins show many anti-angiogenesis effects such as lowering monocyte chemo-attractant protein-1, T-lymphocyte activation, cytokine activity, metalloproteinase, angiotensin-2, pre-proendothelin gene, actin filament, focal adhesion formation, invasiveness, and metastasis spread, along with increased autophagy and endothelial apoptosis, decreased vascular endothelial growth factor (VEGF) receptor-2 activity, and lowered geranyl-geranylated Rho protein release from endothelial cells [3].

2.2 Mechanisms of statin anticancer actions

At molecular level, several clinical studies on nano-based statin use suggested the following altered mechanisms:

Statins inhibit the expression of transcriptional co-activator with PDZ-binding motif (TAZ) on the downstream and LATS1, LATS2, microRNA-9-3p on upstream regions in hepatocellular carcinoma [4]. Statins inhibit the prenylation of Ras superfamily protein. Statins block the MEK/Erk with PI_3K/PKB pathways to arrest the proliferation and growing metastasis [5, 6]. As a result, low PI_3K and poor PKB/AKT activated mTOR downstream expression reduces the small-cell lung cancer cell survival, cell proliferation and motility [7]. Simultaneously, AKT/PKB activated effects such as NFκB-induced PTEN repression, enhanced cyclin D1, COX-2, BCL, survivin, MMP-9 gene-expression disrupt the P-glycoprotein-ATP binding cassette-multidrug resistance protein (PG-ABC-MRP-3) transporter function and increase the drug accumulation in cancer cells. All these statin induced effects suppress the RhoA GTPase activity to induce anti-tumor proliferation and antiapoptosis functions [8]. Statins neutralize the IL-6 induced JAK2/STAT3 pro-inflammatory activation pathway [9]. Stains downregulate the cyclin-dependent CDK1, CDK2, CDK4 with cyclins D1 and cyclin E kinases in Go/G1 phase. Statins upregulate the cyclin-dependent kinase specific p19 and p27 inhibitors [10]. Statins suppress the inflammation to induce the tumor cytotoxic properties. For example, lipophilic simvastatin lowers the geranyl-geranyl pyrophosphate and farnesyl pyrophosphate to trigger the pro-apoptosis, tumor cell growth inhibition to destroy the energy-starved cancer cells in acidic environment. Statins increase the expression of Bax pro-apoptosis factor with a decrease of BCL-2 anti-apoptosis factor expression and high cytochrome C in mitochondrial intrinsic pathway in cells. On other side, cancer cells survive longer by inhibiting the apoptosis.

Pre-clinical studies also support the claim of nano-based statin-reduced low-risks of the deaths from breast, prostate, colorectal cancers by inhibition of endothelial cell proliferation, migration to induce the apoptosis and radiosensitivity in cancer cells [11, 12]. Statins inhibit the tumor uncontrolled cell growth or uncontrolled metastasis. Statins reduce the cancer cell proliferation and survival by c-Jun-N-terminal kinase (JNK) pathways. Thus, active apoptosis inhibits above pathways and reduces the invasion power in cancer cells. Statins upregulate and cluster the Fas-ligands (FasL) on cancer cell surface to activate the caspase-8 and apoptosis in extrinsic pathway.

Statins decrease the metastatic dissemination of tumors and reduce the patient mortality. Several anticancer effects are autophagy, cell death, ferroptosis and pyroptosis. Simvastatin promotes autophagy in cancer cells to inhibit or prevent metastasis spread by adenosine monophosphate-activated protein kinase-target of rapamycin (AMPK-TOR) signal activation. Due to lipophilic nature, simvastatin modifies the epithelial-mesenchymal cell markers and expression pattern of stemness to affect the cancer cell assembly and spheroid formation. Statins regulate the serine/threonine protein kinase Akt that may affect the metastasis. However, in triple-negative breast cancers, statins promote the invasiveness overtime. Statins in combination with chemodrugs show many synergistic effects with reversed multidrug resistance in cancer treatment.

3. Nanocaged statins in combination with chemotherapy and radiotherapy administered in cancer treatment

Second-generation statins at 30–40 mg are given mostly for chemoprevention. Third-generation rosuvastatin at 5–20 mg is the choice in combination therapy. Lovastatin, pravastatin, simvastatin, fluvastatin, atorvastatin, pitavastatin, rosuvastatin, cerivastatin, and mevastatin are given at 20–80 mg/day in combination with chemo-radiotherapy. All statins reduce the cancer resistance by Ras and Rho proteins and modify several biochemical processes. Chemotherapy drugs such as doxorubicine, 5-fluorouracil, paclitaxel, lestaurtinib, capecitabine, sorfenib, gefitinib, erlotinib, imatinib, cisplatin, gemcitabine doxorubicin (~100 M), vemurafenib, and TNF-related apoptosis-inducing ligand (TRAIL) are the ideal choice of anticancer nanocaged drugs to combine with the aforementioned statins (see **Table 1**).

A review is available on statin–chemotherapy combination, highlighting the possibility of nanocaged statins to enhance the following anticancer effects [13]. Another review highlights the nanocaged statins in combination trimodal therapies with a focus on radio-chemodrug action [14]. Our new proposed nano-trimodal therapy is motivated from the following molecular evidences and benefits of nanocaged statins given in combination with chemo-radiotherapy

Nanomaterial/ Nanoparticle	Statin + Chemodrug	Outcome
pH-specific liposome	Simvastatin + doxorubicin	Synergistic effect of SpHL-D-S, reduced cell migration Uterine leiomyoma—No significant change Colon cancer—Pronounced angiogenesis inhibition
Deformed liposome	Vorinostat + simvastatin	Lewis lung cancer—reduced angiogenesis, macrophages, T-cells
Hyaluronan–liposome	Fluvastatin-15 + doxorubicin-3	Breast cancer—Inhibited growth
Liposome	Simvastatin + gefitinib	Lung cancer—Reversed resistance, drug in metastasis
Liposome	Lovastatin + doxorubicin	Liver cancer—Inhibited tumor growth
Herceptin-coated liposome	Simvastatin + doxorubicin	Prostate cancer—Synergistic and angiogenesis effects
Liposome	Simvastatin +5-fluorouracil	Colon cancer—Reduced tumor growth
Hairpin liposome	Simvastatin + paclitaxel	Lung cancer—Reversed epithelial-MSC, macrophages
Immuno-liposome	Simvastatin	Breast cancer—HER2-apoptosis, ERK/AKT/ tumor growth inhibition
Micelle	Simvastatin + Na-Alendronate	3-ve breast/prostate/lung adenocarcinoma—Inhibited tumor growth
Micelle nanoprobe	Simvastatin + ProtoporphyrinIX	Glioma—Cell cycle G1-S phase arrest, high apoptosis/reactive oxygen
Micelle	Atorvastatin	Glioblastoma/glioma—Inhibited cancer growth, high drug in tumor
Nanoemulsion—lipids	Atorvastatin	Intestinal cancer—Inhibited tumor growth
Nanoemulsion—lipids	Doxorubicin + pravastatin	Ehrlich ascites carcinoma—Increased survival Breast cancer, foreskin cancer—Reduced cytotoxicity and side effects
Nanoemulsion	Simvastatin + doxorubicin	Ehrlich ascites carcinoma—Reduced cytotoxicity
Lipid nanoparticles	Atorvastatin	Breast cancer—Increased bioavailability, growth inhibition
ChitosanEudragit-S100	Simvastatin	Colon cancer—Reduced cytotoxicity, arrested G2/M phase
Chitosan-TGP PR-CNG-ER	Simvastatin	Breast cancer—High entrapment, controlled growth Liver cancer—Better entrapment, drug loading, two-day sustained release
SVCSChS-NPs	Simvastatin, ASPGR	Hepatocellular carcinoma—Inhibited proliferation, high cell uptake
PEG/lipids(Labrafil/ Labrafac)	Simvastatin	Breast cancer—High cell viability in presence of Labrafil/Labrafac
PLGA-PEG-MAN	Simvastatin	HCC—Alleviated LSEC capillarization, regressed stroma, NO signaling
PCL-PEG-PCL	Atorvastatin + rosuvastatin	Breast cancer—Inhibited growth, high cytotoxicity
PCL-PEG	Simvastatin	Breast cancer—Sustained drug release, dose-specific growth inhibition

Nanomaterial/ Nanoparticle	Statin + Chemodrug	Outcome
PCL-PEG	Simvastatin +5-fluorouracil	Gastric cancer—Induced apoptosis, autophagy, low metastsis
PLGA micron NP	Simvastatin	Breast cancer solid tumors—High AUC,$T_{1/2}$,C_{max}, low K_{el}
PLGA	Simvastatin + gemcitabine	Pancreatic/breast cancers—High bioavailability/cytotoxicity, low IC_{50} value

Table 1.
Statin-loaded chemo-radiotherapy nanoformulations made of liposomes, micelles, emulsions, and polymers used in clinical research.

and/or immunotherapy, targeted therapy, and others in cancer treatment [15]. The major benefit is the user-friendly nanomaterial cage as a safe delivery carrier to offer minimal damage to surrounding normal cells from chemo-radiotherapy given with statins.

3.1 Statin-induced apoptosis and autophagy

Simvastatin is the most cited statin [16]. In general, statin shows tumor suppressor action. Statins likely induce the cancer cell apoptosis through depletion of isoprenoid-protein prenylation enabled low geranyl-geranyl PP and Ras/Rho GTPase that modifies the membrane and cell signaling. Such depleted c-Jun expression and cdk2, E2F1, p21/p27, and Bcl-2/elevated Bax protein changes trigger the mislocalization and protein malfunctioning for programmed cell death or apoptosis. Statins show synergistic effects. For example, fluvastatin activates the AMPK-mTOR protein while lovastatin suppresses the cancer cell viability via inducing autophagy in cancers of ovary and lung, malignant pleural mesothelioma, pancreatic cancer, and melanoma [17].

3.2 Chemotherapy and radiotherapy

Both these chemodrug–EBRT radiation therapies generate the ROS species. In nanocages, the statins may minimize the ROS damage to normal cells. These cytotoxic ROS species induce the following effects:

- Oxidative stress, endothelial dysfunction, inflammation, and fibrosis in normal cells
- DNA damage, lipid peroxidation, protein nitrosylation, and inhibition of IRS/PI3K/Akt pathways with enhanced MAPK-induced signaling pathway after radiation therapy-induced water decomposition in cancer cells
- Low NO bioavailability-induced ET1 production, endothelial dysfunction, inflammation, thrombosis, and fibrosis
- Activated NF-kB upregulation of cytokine expression, and NF-kB targeting the adhesion factors to promote acute inflammation

- TGF-β induced vascular fibrosis (collagen and ECM accumulation) or lumen narrowing
- Mitochondrial damage.

In combination, nanocaged chemo-radiotherapy induces the immune response to kill immunogenic tumor cells effectively by the use of immunotherapy, sparing the normal cells with least toxicity.

3.3 Immunotherapy

Nanocaged statins may minimize the adverse effects of the enhanced immune regulation by CAR-T cell therapy (chimeric protein activated cell to destroy the surface target antigens) and ICI therapies (immune attack of antibodies activating T-cell protein-4, PD-1 and PD-1 ligand). Immunotherapy with statins reduces the cancer-induced cardiovascular complications of endothelial dysfunction, atherosclerosis plaque, myocarditis, arrhythmia, heart failure, thrombosis, vasculitis, thromboembolism, and others. These immunotherapies are available as tumor vaccines, oncolytic viruses, immuno-adjuvants, check-point inhibitors, and cellular immunotherapies.

3.4 Antiproliferative therapy

Nanocaged statins may minimize the toxic effects of antineoplastic chemodrug-suppressed proliferation via STAT/SKP2 signaling, Wnt signaling (AT-rich binding protein-1 regulation), TAZ down-regulation, DNA methyltransferase inhibition (epigenetic changes), stem cell differentiation, and YAP/CD144 growth axis.

3.5 Targeted therapy

Nanocaged statins may minimize the toxic effects of targeted therapies such as oxidative stress, mitochondrial damage and apoptosis directed at human epidermal receptor-2 (HER-2) or ERBB2/ERBB4 receptors, MAPK/ERK kinase (MEK), vascular endothelial growth VEGF receptor, BCR-ABL kinase activity. Trastuzumab does TKI-targeting the VEGF and MEK signal pathways.

3.6 Antioxidant therapy

Nanocaged statins may reduce the ROS species by down-regulation of NADPH-Oxidase-1 RNA to stop Rac-1 translocation to cell membrane (NoX-1 and ROS inhibition) and Keap-1/Nrf-2 signal pathways.

3.7 Anti-angiogenesis therapy

Nanocaged cerevastatin inhibits RhoA/focal adhesion kinase/Akt pathways. Nanocaged simvastatin with bevacizumab inhibits RhoA geranyl–geranylation and improves colorectal cancer. Nanocaged atorvastatin may down-regulate both VEGF and CD31 expressions. Nanocaged rosuvastatin reduces angiogenesis. All these events show anti-angiogenesis.

3.8 Anti-inflammatory therapy

Nanocaged simvastatin may inhibit the Rho GTPase and NF-kB translocation required for ICAMs, VCAMs, RhoA, Rac1, and Cdc42 inflammatory molecules. Nanocaged atorvastatin reduces the NF-kB transcription by MAPK signal ERK, JNK, and p38 pathways in the presence of PPARγ activation.

3.9 Antifibrotic therapy

Nanocaged statins may hinder the Rho/Ras-ERK-1/2 pathway and decrease the collagen expression and fibroblast proliferation by activation of AMPK and down-regulation of TGF-β/SMAD-2 or – 3/CTGF pathways to mitigate the fibroblast ECM fibrosis and myocardial hypertrophy.

3.10 Metastasis prevention therapy

Limited use of nanocaged pravastatin and simvastatin may prevent the skeletal metastasis of breast cancer by inhibition of CD44 expression or enhancing the p53 expression. However, meta-analysis indicated that statins reduce the risk of prostate cancer metastasis.

3.11 Antisense therapy

Nanocaged statins may induce the short interfering RNA (siRNA), antisense oligonucleotide (ASO), and hypoxia-inducible factor (HIF) to mitigate the immunosuppression, tumor angiogenesis, multidrug resistance, photodynamic therapy resistance, and metastasis [18].

4. Statin-loaded nanoformulation design

The triple-modal nanomedicine as nanocaged statin combined with chemo-radiotherapy, immunotherapy, and/or targeted therapy agents mainly reduces the normal cell cytotoxicity and controls the anticancer metabolic regulation by altering tumor cell gene regulation proteins. Also, nanomedicine minimizes the barriers of membrane transport channels or uptake gates for unrestricted controlled release of statins and/or chemo-radiotherapy drugs out of their nanocarrier coating for prolonged stay of drugs in the tumor microenvironment.

Two major methods of nanoformulations are (1) the top-down nanomilling/wet milling method of mechanical force to reduce statin particle size, and the high-pressure homogenization method to force statin dispersion through a small nozzle for making nano-sized particles; and (2) the bottom-up solvent evaporation method of statin–chitosan mix in solvent and its second evaporation to make nanoparticles, another lipid melt-emulsification with surfactant ultrasonication method to make solid lipid nanoparticles, the microfluidic mixing method to create monodisperse statin-loaded nanoparticles with controlled size and properties, and sustainable methods to replace toxic organic solvents with polyethylene glycol to prepare statin-loaded nanoparticles.

Nanocaged statin nanoplatforms have high loading capacity, good delivery, cell uptake, and efficient statin encapsulation. Statin-chemodrug nanoparticle size is in the range of 60–90 nm, and they have high surface charge or high zeta potential, stable structure, good drug release profile, and effectiveness in cell cultures and tumors.

Nanotechnology enhances the targeted delivery of statins and/or immuno-chemodrugs to specific tissues or cancer cells with improved efficacy and minimal side effects. The nanoformulation is designed to co-deliver statins slowly with controlled release of chemotherapeutic agents to enhance the radiosensitizing effects. Specific examples are microfluidic mixed HDL–liposomes loaded with simvastatin to enhance the radiosensitization in head–neck squamous cell carcinoma, melt-emulsification-ultrasonicated solid lipid nanoparticles loaded with atorvastatin, and sustainable PEGylation of statin with PEG 400 or PLGA to encapsulate statins in cancer treatment.

A review of different nanoformulation methods is available for use in preclinical trials [18]. Still, the wider use of nanoformulations in clinical practice is awaited.

4.1 Benefits of statin-loaded nanoplatforms

Very little data is available on growing demand for the triple modal hybrid nanodelivery method, but several clinical studies indicate the benefits of nanoplatforms for statins combined with other therapies as follows.

- European Society of Cardiology cardio-oncology guidelines recommend statins for primary prevention by nanodelivery in patients at high risk of anthracycline-induced cardiotoxicity (Grade IIa, Level of Evidence B) [19].

- A retrospective case-control study (n = 628) women with breast cancer receiving anthracycline with atorvastatin in nanocage showed a reduced risk of heart failure, LVEF [20, 21].

- Another observational radomized control trial (RCT) study (n = 300) on lymphoma reduced the cardiac dysfunction [22].

- A retrospective analysis (n = 478) on non-small-cell lung cancer (NSCLC) patients undergoing curative-intent (chemo) radiotherapy revealed that high-intensity or moderate statin therapy by nanodelivery is more beneficial before radiation therapy to NSCLC. It reduces the need for a radiation dose (>3 Gy) in existing Cardiovascular disease (CVD) patients with risk factors of CVD to improve their overall survival [23].

- A retrospective analysis (n = 748) of locally advanced NSCLC patients receiving controlled and restricted thoracic radiation therapy showed that statins are inversely associated with survival rate [24]. This indicates that statin treatment reduces cardiotoxicity, but statin-induced high cardiovascular risk factors demand safe statin delivery and longer stay. It remains to be explored if prolonged stay of statins in tumor may have any additional cardioprotective role on chemo-radiotherapy-induced or radiation-induced cardiotoxicities with comprehensive evaluation of the baseline cardiac risk after cardiac radiation dose exposure.

- A retrospective study of 129 HER2-positive breast cancer patients on trastuzumab treatment showed that patients treated with prolonged stay of statins in nanocarriers had 68% lower odds of cardiotoxicity [25].

- A retrospective study on females aged 70+ years with breast cancer showed that statin combined with trastuzumab treatment could not avoid the heart failure [26].

5. Statins and trimodal nanotherapies

Trimodal statin loaded with chemo-radiotherapy–immunotherapy or radiation therapy agents demands a specific different set of physical and chemical properties of biologicals (robotic navigator–tumor killer–alert performer) used in nanoformulation design such as the following.

- Nano-based lipid or polymer-based statin delivery systems to improve solubility, stability, bioavailability, and target tumor statin delivery.

- Nanosystems to deliver and protect statins as stable therapeutic, less toxic, circulating nanoformulations in the bloodstream with no side effects.

- Different polymers of chitosan, PEG, PCI, PGLA and liposomes, nanoemulsions, nanomicelles to offer options of nanocarriers to gold nanoshells, nanorods, iron oxide nanoparticles with therapeutic potentials in breast cancer, prostate cancer, brain glioblastoma, and liver cancer. Different nanoassemblies are used in the following nanoformulations.

5.1 Lipid-based liposomes

Statin-loaded liposomes are biocompatible and biodegradable phospholipids. They encapsulate and deliver the hydrophilic statins stored in core or hydrophobic statins stored in the lipid bilayer as a flexible drug delivery system. Liposomes encapsulate statins with chemo-radiotherapy and/or immunotherapy agents. Liposomes reduce drug toxicity on healthy cells with no side effects. Liposomes bind to ligands and functionalize them as antibodies or active targeting cancer cell receptor-bound peptides to enhance the permeability and retention effects across leaky tumor vasculature. However, liposomes aggregate and degrade fast with less drug-loading capacity. So, PEGylation of liposomes is a design option of stable liposomes to provoke immune responses and to deliver photosensitizers in cancer cell killing. For example, nanoformulation of liposome action facilitates the passive targeting or Doxil® chemodrug accumulation in tumor vasculature [27]. Liposome hyaluronan-encapsulated simvastatin or fluvastatin combined with doxorubicin in ratio 1:2 improves the doxorubicin delivery to enhance its antiproliferative effect and antitumor response in tumor macrophage M2 → repolarized M1 tumor phenotype-rich environment (intratumor infiltration ability) of colon cancer [27]. Liposome encapsulated combinations of simvastatin–gefitinib increases the drug penetration with minimum drug resistance by elevated ROS and suppressed EGFR/Akt/Erk signaling pathway [28]. Other examples of statin-loaded liposomes are herceptin-conjugated encapsulating doxorubicin–simvastatin for prostate cancer; flurouracil–simvastatin in colon cancer; paclitaxel–simvastatin in epithelial–mesenchymal transition reversion; and anti-HER2 loaded immunoliposome–simvastatin in breast cancer cells overexpressing HER2 [28]. These liposome combinations target the highly selected HER2-overexpressing breast cancers with least-nonspecific cytotoxicity.

5.2 Micelles

Small-sized micelle-based nanocarriers enhance the hydrophobic drug solubility, accumulation, and tumor penetrability. Micelles can bind to targeting ligands on surface and can be PEGylated to enhance the circumventing time within tumor and specific drug targets. However, micelles have less space for drug encapsulation, are less stable in tumor and bloodstream, show less drug loading capacity or premature drug release, and are less effective. Nanomicelles encapsulating hydrophobic paclitaxel and doxorubicin with simvastatin are small-sized particles with large surface to enhance drug accumulation characteristics. Statins in nanocarriers are used to combat multidrug resistance in tumors. These nanomicelles also encapsulate chemotherapeutics and signaling inhibitors to influence synergistic effects in cancer treatment. Examples include the following:

- Simvastatin with Na-alendronate to arrest cell cycle as a pro-apoptotic, tumor cytotoxic agent to inhibit cell growth with low IC50 values and inhibit multiplication in S phase
- Nanomicelles that release simvastatin and protoporphyrin IX after light irradiation to trigger reactive oxygen species (ROS) with synergistic apoptosis necrosis to arrest cell cycle
- Nanomicelles encapsulated atorvastatin to enhance blood-brain-barrier permeability and glioblastoma tumor cytotoxicity

5.3 Nanoemulsions

Oil-in-water nanoemulsions enhance solubility and bioavailability of hydrophobic statin as long-term drug-loaded stores with thermodynamic stability and prolonged drug delivery applications. However, nanoemulsions are rapidly cleared by the reticuloendothelial system. So, nanoemulsions have poor circulation time, restricted targeting capability, and poor functionalization with targeting ligands such as high risk of emulsifying surfactant toxicity in skin cancer. Examples are as follows:

- Author reported nanocurcumin with lipophilic paclitaxel as a combination cancer drug [29].
- Atorvastatin-loaded nano-anchor (deoxycholic acid-DTMP-biotin-tocopherol-PEG succinate) increases the oral atorvastatin bioavailability and suppresses tumor growth [30].
- Nanoemulsion gel carrier of lovastatin-loaded eucalyptus oil drug delivery system showed synergistic effects and inhibition of tongue cancer [31].
- Nanoemulsion of paravastatin with doxorubicin reduce drug toxicity in heart and liver tissues [32].
- Simvastatin and pravastatin with doxorubicin showed antitumor activity against Ehrlich ascites carcinoma and breast cancer with more efficiency [33].
- Lipid-based drug delivery nanoemulsions are safe with high surface area and enhanced permeability and retention (EPR); are nontoxic, stable, and

biodegradable; and offer least leakage from stored or circulating controlled drug release carriers for long-term cancer treatment and preventing siRNA or DNA from enzyme degradation with sustained therapeutic effects [34].

However, all these efficient hydrophobic nanoemulsions restrict encapsulating hydrophilic drug loading and delivery because of optimal surfactant lipid composition and particle size requirements. In cancer therapy, the author reviewed lipid-based nanoparticle-based delivery of siRNA and mRNA combined with chemodrugs precisely to target oncogenes or chemotherapy and modulate immune responses [35]. Examples are (1) glycerol monostearate encapsulated atorvastatin with vinpocetine in breast, melanoma, and liver cancer therapy [36]; and (2) atorvastatin-loaded GMS-stearate-carnauba wax nanoparticles in MCF-7 breast cancer cells [37].

5.4 Polymer nanocarriers

Polymer-based nanoformulations are chitosan, polyethylene glycol, poly-lactic co-glycollate (PLGA) conjugated with possible lovastatin, paravastatin, rosuvastatin, atorvastatin, simvastatin, or chemodrugs and superparamagnetic iron oxide agents. Chitosan, derived from crustaceans, is highly biodegradable and biocompatible, with antioxidant, antibacterial, antitumor, high cancer cell uptake, and selective tumor permeability properties to induce apoptosis, and it inhibits the tumor cell proliferation or survival by enzyme actions and its antiangiogenic gene expression modulation [38].

5.4.1 Chitosan nanoformulations

Chitosan-encapsulated, statin-loaded nanocarriers, with active amino, acetamido, and hydroxyl groups, protect the statins and facilitate pH-dependent sustained drug release to deliver them efficiently at ensured tumor site with maximum efficacy, enhanced solubility and anticancer activity, and least toxicity. Examples include the following:

- Eudragit S100 chitosan–iron oxide based simvastatin is used for targeting and cytotoxicity against colon cancer HCT-116 cells [39].
- Chitosan-coated simvastatin nanoparticles inhibit proliferation of tongue carcinoma HSC-3 cells [40].
- Poloxamer188 with chitosan face-centered-central (FCC) composite to precipitate and dope simvastatin with quercetin (SIM-QRC) nanoparticles enhanced apoptosis viacaspase-3 and tumor suppressor proteins [41].
- Chitosan-tamarind gum polysaccharide polyelectrolyte-coated simvastatin complex stabilizes small-sized nanoparticles with high statin entrapment against breast cancer [42].
- Chicken egg and tomato peel membrane also had pro-apoptosis activity against tumor growth [43].

- Erythrocytes loaded with chitosan-pravastatin nanogels (PR-CNG-ER) exposed to phosphatidylserine showed stomatocyte, high entrapping efficiency, and antiproliferative activity for liver cancer treatments [44].

- cross-linked tripolyphosphate chondroitin sulfate with simvastatin nanoparticles enhanced oral bioavailability and safe asialoglycoprotein receptor mediated delivery to inhibit proliferation and enhanced cellular uptake endocytosis against hepatocellular carcinoma [45].

5.4.2 Polyethylene glycol nanoformulations

A polyethylene glycol (PEG) based nanodrug delivery system improves the hydrophobic drug solubility and stability to increase the statin bioavailability. PEGylation is a process to attach hydrophilic PEG chains to statins that prolongs statin circulation time or slow clearance from blood (stealthness) by evading immune detection across the nanocage surface to enhance the controlled and sustained pH-dependent drug release, biodistribution, pharmacokinetics, permeability, accumulation, and retention at the tumor site with no toxicity [46]. Recently, our team has developed PEGylated Cas-IFN nanoparticles that bind with ligands and functionalize to deliver statins directly into cancer cells and enhance statin solubility, prolong circulation time, and offer low immunogenicity, controlled drug delivery, high therapeutic efficacy or minimum toxicity to healthy cells, and off-target effects as ideal for safe, effective cancer therapies. Other examples are as follows:

- Simvastatin release across oleoyl-macrogel-6-glycerides (Labrasol ®M1944 CS), caprylocaproylmacrogol-8-glycerides (Labrafac lipophile® WL1349) nanolipid carriers in PBS pH 7.4 was used for nontoxic antitumor activity [47]

- Nanodelivery of PEGylated simvastatin targeted the liver sinusoidal endothelial cells in fibrotic HCC patients showing low capillarization and suppressed tumor growth [48]

- Polycaprolactone (PCL) with PEG copolymer biodegradable nanomicelle is used as an atorvastatin/rosuvastatin carrier to enhance the statin loading, kinetic release, cytotoxicity, and anticancer activity for breast cancer treatment [49].

- Simvastatin polycaprolactone–polyethylene glycol (SMV-PCL-PEG) nanocarrier enhanced dose-dependent cytotoxicity and sub-G1 cell populations, lowered 5-flurouracil resistance, and increased apoptosis and autophagy in gastric cancer or metastasis [50].

5.4.3 Poly lactic-Co-glycolic acid (PGLA) nanoformulations

Biodegradable PGLA polymers are biocompatible with controlled drug delivery. These sustained-release systems enhance the statin solubility and stability. These statin-loaded PGLAs functionalize with targeting ligands to further improve the statin delivery, boosting efficiency with least side effects. Examples are as follows:

- Simvastatin-loaded PGLA submicron nanospray particles facilitate the high drug loading and formulation yield (large area under the curve), terminal half-life, and plasma concentration or low elimination rate constant [51].

- Simvastatin and PGLA-gemcitabine (SMV-PGLA-GM) encapsulated nanoparticles improved bioavailability, inhibited proliferative activity, and offered better absorption and systemic residence [52].
- Simvastatin and miRNA conjugated PLGA/PEI nanoparticles enhanced the apoptosis and therapeutic efficacy with least cytotoxicity in gastric cancer [53].

5.4.4 Hybrid organic-inorganic nanoformulations

Several organic–inorganic nanoparticles enhance the statin-based chemodrug controlled delivery and sustained statin release to target the tumors with a low statin dose. These hybrid nanoparticles bind to targeting ligands that functionalize for safe statin delivery to cancer cells and minimize off-target effects for theranosis. Examples are as follows:

- Simvastatin conjugated poly lactic-co-glycolic acid (SMV-PLGA) combined with superparamagnetic iron oxide (SPION) nanoparticles enhances the apoptosis and reduces necrosis in prostate cancer [54].
- Simvastatin conjugated chitosan lipid carriers (SMV-Ch-NLCs) enhanced statin release, skin permeation, uptake, adhesion, and effectiveness with inhibited proliferation and cell growth in melanoma treatment [55].
- Carboxylated graphene oxide (CGO)–trimethyl chitosan–hyaluronate and chitosan conjugated TPGS-b-(PCL-ran-PGA) nanoparticles enhanced HIF-1 α siRNA or oligonucleotide release into nasopharyngeal carcinoma cells to reduce the chemoresistance of carcinoma cells by down-regulation of HIF-1-α [56].

The nanoformulations may reduce the tumor multidrug resistance of hypoxic cancer cells via reducing abundant reactive oxygen species under X-ray irradiation. These nanoformulations inhibit the HIF-1α expression and disturb the self-restoration of impaired double-stranded DNA. Gold nanocomposites deliver the HIF-1-α siRNA and significantly improve the radiation sensitivity of hypoxic nasopharyngeal carcinoma cells [57].

6. Physician's guide

In cancer therapy, physicians aim to achieve statin-induced cholesterol-lowering and effectively reduced cardiotoxicity or cardiac protection with statin-induced apoptosis, inhibited angiogenesis, modulated autophagy, reduced risks of metastasis, and modulated tumor environment to overcome the chemodrug resistance and enhance overall survival [58].

Simvastatin is an excellent choice as a tumor suppressor. Statins are mostly prescribed in low 5–20 mg or moderate 20–40 mg doses to induce apoptosis (through traditional NFkB, inhibiting canonical caspase cascades and proliferation through MEK1/2, FRK1/2, and JNK pathways). At high statin dose of 80–100 mg, different statins induce cell cycle arrest (by p21/p16 protein/DNMTs through AMPK activation and increased p21 and p27), expression, migration, cancer cell invasion (by pituitary tumor-transforming gene-1 [PTTG1] suppression), epithelial–mesenchymal transition (EMT), and chemoresistance in breast, lung, pancreas, and liver cancers. A representative physician's guide of different statin doses was prescribed to achieve benefits of co-therapies [17].

Different nanomaterials used to reduce the cardiotoxicity and chance of avoiding heart failure among patients treated by statin-loaded nanoformulations with combined chemo-radiotherapy and/or immunotherapy agents are as shown in **Table 1**.

The recent clinical trials suggest different anticancer statin benefits with evidence as shown in **Table 2**.

Clinical Study	Anticancer Drugs with Statins		Patient Outcome	Ref
Retrospective case-control study in BC (n = 628)	Anthracycline	Atorvastatin	Incident HF and cancer-related low mortality in statin group	[20]
Retrospective study in BC, ALL, lymphoma (n = 51)	Anthracycline	Simvastatin, atorvastatin	Decreased LVEF by anthracyclines	[59]
Random-control trial (n = 40)	Anthracycline	Atorvastatin	Maintained LVEF by anthracyclines	[60]
Double-blind random-control trial on lymphoma (n = 300)	Anthracycline chemotherapy	Atorvastatin	Reduced cardiac dysfunction by anthracyclines	[22]
Retrospective analysis in NSCLC patients (n = 478)	Chemo-radiotherapy	Different statins	Enhanced NSCL patient survival	[24]
Retrospective case-control study on HER2 + ve breast cancer patients (n = 525)	Trastuzumab therapy	Atorvastatin, rosuvastatin, simvastatin, pravastatin	Low risk of cardiotoxicity	[61]
Single center study	ICI	Statins	ICI reduced atheroplaques	[62]
NCT06241352	Chemotherapy	Atorvastatin	Advanced Pancreatic cancer	NIH
NCT03971019	EBRT	Simvastatin	Breast cancer survival	NIH
NCT04601116 (MASTER)	Chemodrug	Atorvastatin	ER + ve patient survival	NIH
NCT03024684 (SHOT)	Curative therapy	Atorvastatin	HCC recurrence/ prevents	NIH
NCT04457089	Platinum	Simvastatin	Ovarian cancer low progression	NIH
NCT05696973 (MOVES)	Exercise	Atorvastatin	Onco-exercise	NIH
NCT03560882 (Pilot p53)	Chemodrug	Atorvastatin	P53 M/W malignancy	NIH
NCT03889795 (Phase IB)	Metformin + digoxin	Simvastatin	Solid tumors	NIH
NCT06030622 (Phase 2A-C3)	Metformin + Digoxin	Simvastatin	Recurrent/refractory pancreatic cancer (C3)	NIH
NCT05550415	—	Simvastatin	Epithelial mesenchymal transition	NIH

Clinical Study	Anticancer Drugs with Statins		Patient Outcome	Ref
NCT05977738 (ReDiReCCT-P)	Calcium	Pitavastatin	Breast, prostate cancers	NIH
NCT04767984	Calcium	Atorvastatin	Colon cancer + ulcerative colitis	NIH
NCT04491643	Megestrol acetate	Rosuvastatin	Early endometrial carcinoma	NIH

Abbreviation: NIH – http://www.grants.gov/.

Table 2.
Clinical trial studies on statin-loaded chemo-radiotherapy with enhanced patient outcome.

Some major onco-therapeutic benefits and challenges of statin chemo-radiotherapy are as follows:

- Lovastatin and pravastatin reduce metastasis through the RhoA signal. Lovastatin and atorvastatin induce apoptosis (through the JNK/Rac1/Cdc42 pathway) and autophagy (by AMPK/Akt/mTOR pathways). Atorvastatin, lovastatin, fluvastatin, and simvastatin combined with doxorubicin are ideal to induce apoptosis. However, simvastatin combined with paclitaxel stops tumor growth [63].

- High doses of statins reduce the cancer risk but may cause mitochondrial toxicity such as myopathies (by inhibited respiratory chain complex, induced apoptosis, Q10 reduction, Ca^{++} metabolic dysregulation, and CPT-2 enzyme expression). Care is needed to manage diabetes along with dementia and myopathies [64].

- Statins with chemoradiotherapy reduce cardiotoxicity in breast cancer. Preferred hydrophilic rosuvastatin and pravastatin reduce the adverse cardiovascular risks [65].

- Atorvastatin prolonged use at high dose effectively reduces radiation-induced fibrosis while lovastatin in high doses enhances radiation-induced apoptosis [66].

- Statins reduce resistance. Statins as single monotherapy are preferred as an apoptosis inducer and antiproliferative choice. In combination with chemodrugs, statins reduce resistance by synergistic action [13].

- Fluvastatin and atorvastatin combined with chemodrugs are smart antiproliferative, anti-cytotoxicity, cell cycle progress (activation in G0/G1 with inhibition in S phase and G2/M phase), and ERK MAP kinase transduction activation approaches to reduce aggressive leukemia spread [67].

- Rosuvastatin is an excellent choice for reducing rectal cancer risk in combination with neo-adjuvant chemo-radiation (NACTRT) for better pathology response pCR rates [68].

- Statins mitigate cardiotoxicity.

- Lipophilic 20 mg statins (lovastatin, simvastatin, fluvastatin, atorvastatin) and hydrophilic statins (pravastatin and rosuvastatin), combined with cholesterol absorption inhibitor ezetimbe 10 mg, enhance the cytochrome P450 isoenzyme and statin clearance by kidney and liver, respectively. However, monotherapy shows adverse effects of upper respiratory infection (URI), diarrhea, sinusitis, arthralgia, nasopharyngitis, myalgia, and stroke in post-radiotherapy cancer patients [69].

- Both hydrophilic and lipophilic statins reduce the toxicity from radiotherapy in ENT but show hepatitis, transaminitis, myopathy, myositis/myalgia, sleep disorders, and rhabdomyolysis as side effects [70].

- Fluvastatin 200 mg/kg wt and simvastatin 180 mg/kg wt doses suppress tumor by 80.5 and 58.5%, respectively, but enhance cytotoxic/cytostatic chemo-resistance anticancer effects [17].

- Lovastatin and mevastatin implementation inhibits carcinogenesis and contributes radiosensitization during late G1 and G2-M cell cycle phases after radiation treatment with better clinical outcome benefits in prostate cancer. Safely, statins can be given to inactivate RhoA and cyclooxygenase-2 [71].

- Rosuvastatin is the best choice. Simvastatin and pravastatin combined with concurrent chemo-radiotherapy enhanced the overall survival benefits in a dose-dependent fashion to treat esophagus cancer [72].

- Simvastatin combined with radiotherapy dose prevented mitochondria in advanced small-cell lung cancer clinical trials and improved 5-year survival rates by 20% [73].

- Statin-induced chemotherapy with radiotherapy or chemo-radiotherapy (CCRT) effectively reduced toxicity in nasopharyngeal carcinoma with survival of 76 months and grade 3 to 4 short-term toxic effects [74].

- Statins combined with radiation doses may reduce the risk of volumetric modulated arc therapy (VMAT) or intensity modulated radiation therapy (IMRT) radiation-induced cardiotoxicity. Different cardiovascular indicators (hypertension, dyslipidemia, diabetes, QRISK score, coronary artery disease (CAD)/cardiovascular disease (CVD), arrhythmia, heart failure, peripheral vascular disease, aneurysm, valvulopathy, and treatments) may evaluate the overall outcomes [23].

- Low-dose simvastatin neoadjuvant therapy combined with fluorouracil, Adriamycin, and cyclophosphamide therapy is recommended to enhance the objective response rate (ORR) in both cancer types: (1) Luminal A: esterogen receptor/progesterone receptor+ve, HER2-ve, Ki-67 < 14%; and (2) Luminal B: HER2 –ve:ER/PR + ve, HER2-ve, Ki-67 > 14%; HER2 + ve:ER/PR + ve, any Ki-67, HER+ve; HER2 + ve:ER/PR absent, HER2 + ve; Triple-ve:ER/PR absent, HER2-ve. However, adverse events also do occur [75].

- Fluvastatin and atorvastatin combined with chemotherapy <20 Gy inhibits proliferation and cytotoxicity of natural killer cell leukemia to enhance overall survival at 20.4–48 months [67].

- Rituzumab, cyclophosphamide, doxorubicine, vincristine, prednisone (R-CHOP) loaded with statins in elderly patients aged >75 years enhance the chemo-chop stage III–IV "double hit" large B-cell lymphoma clinopathologic characteristics [76].

Physicians need to be aware of statins' dark side in making a choice. Statins given as adjuvants in anti-neoplastic treatment may make aggressive malignant tumors more vulnerable. Statins may develop statin intolerance symptoms of muscle pain, stiffness, cramps, exertion, myopathy, mitochondrial toxicity symptoms, and multidrug resistance of mitoxantrone, etoposide, and cyclosporine–pravastatin cytotoxicity.

7. Future prospectives

Conventional antiparasitic, antimalarial and anti-inflammatory drugs (same as statins) combined with lonafarnib may serve as repurposed anti-inflammatory and anticancer nanoformulations in ovarian cancer and gynecological cancers [77]. New nanoformulations will enhance the safe delivery and monitoring of statin effects combined with chemo-radiotherapy, or hybrid trimodal therapy, outcomes in cancer treatment. New nanomaterials will serve as a more effective lipid metabolism-biocompatible encapsulated loading of statins [78] with chemo-radiotherapy and/or immunotherapy, targeting agents within the tumor microenvironment as multipurpose robotic–navigator–nano-alert-performer (RNNAP) nanoformulation particles with better solubility, stability, and tumor-targeting ability (recorded biosensing of pH-dependent tumor-killing) with maximum accumulated anticancer drug concentration in tumor cells with the least systemic side effects. All these measures will reduce chemoradiotherapy toxicities with improved treatment outcomes. Major developments will be as follows:

- Enhanced nanodrug delivery with least damage to healthy tissues and nanotargeting of the tumor cells by nanoparticle surface modification with targeting ligands, utilizing enhanced permeability and retention EPR effect.

- Reducing the chemodrug or radiation therapy resistance by newly explored mechanisms such as overexpression of drug efflux pumps or altered apoptotic pathways. Better nanoparticles or nanoformulations will be engineered to reduce resistance by drug delivery with a better understanding of their anticancer mechanisms and accumulated chemodrugs in tumors.

- New statins combined with chemo-radiotherapy nanoformulations will enhance the synergistic effects, which means a more effective combination therapy than any other treatment alone. Next-generation statins will be better modulating tumor microenvironment with enhanced chemotherapy or radiation effectiveness or targeting tumor growth and survival.

- New nanoformulations will be better statin–chemo-radiotherapy drug delivery platforms with minimal side effects of chemo-radiotherapy for improved patient outcomes and quality of life.

- New designs of nanoparticles will be available for versatile applications such as carriers of multiple chemotherapeutic drugs, radiation sensitizers, and immune-modulating agents for personalized cancer treatment.

- Better nanoparticle-assisted imaging and real-time monitoring of chemodrug delivery and treatment response will be available to clinicians to optimize treatment strategy and personalize patient care.

With the foregoing potentials, the use of nanotechnology still has challenges. However, future directions mainly are focused on the following:

1. Development of scalable and cost-effective nanoparticle manufacturing methods and wider use of nanoparticles in clinics and clinical applications [79, 80].

2. Evaluation of long-term safety and toxicity of nanoformulations used in nanoparticle-based therapies [81, 82].

3. Large-scale multicentric clinical trials to evaluate the efficacy and safety of statin-loaded nanoformulations in cancer patients.

4. Due to no information available on permitted doses of nanocaged chemo-radiotherapy or radiation exposure to normal cells, it needs radiation or radioprotection measures [83].

8. Conclusion

Statins combined with chemodrugs and/or radiotherapy agents can be loaded within nanocarrier platforms for prolonged stay. For statins in combination with chemodrugs and radiotherapy agents, the statins are designed in nanoformulations. Statin-loaded nanoformulations induce better lipid-lowering and anticancer pleiotropic effects to reduce chemo-radiotherapy toxicity with minimal side effects. Different nanoformulations show potentials of better statin delivery and effective statin-induced anticancer mechanisms of cancer treatment. Nanotechnology has given an opportunity of complex nanoformulation design using new options of PEG, PGLA, chitosan, liposomes, micelle, and Qdot to load statins along with chemo-radiotherapy and/or other adjuvant therapies. Triple modal statin–chemo-radiotherapy with other adjuvant therapies serves to get maximum outcomes with least side effects in cancer treatment. However, these techniques are still in infancy with many challenges.

Acknowledgements

The author acknowledges the collaborative efforts of Professor Yuvraj Negi at the Indian Institute of Technology Roorkee; Dr. Shashi Prabha Singh, Government Medical College, Mirzapur; and Professor Yashwant Pathak at University of Central Florida, Tampa for motivation and discussions. The author used AI tools to polish the language and correct interpretation of the concepts in this chapter.

Author details

Rakesh Sharma
Government Medical College, Saharanpur, Uttar Pradesh, India

*Address all correspondence to: rksz2009@gmail.com

References

[1] Siegel RL, Miller KD, Wagle NS, Jemal A. Cancer statistics, 2023. CA: A Cancer Journal for Clinicians. 2023;**73**(1):17-48

[2] Piccolo S, Cordenonsi M, Dupont S. Molecular pathways: YAP and TAZ take center stage in organ growth and tumorigenesis. Clinical Cancer Research. 2013;**19**(18):4925-4930

[3] Sorrentino G, Ruggeri N, Specchia V, Cordenonsi M, Mano M, Dupont S, et al. Metabolic control of YAP and TAZ by the mevalonate pathway. Nature Cell Biology. 2014;**16**(4):357-366

[4] Higashi T, Hayashi H, Kitano Y, Yamamura K, Kaida T, Arima K, et al. Statin attenuates cell proliferative ability via TAZ (WWTR1) in hepatocellular carcinoma. Medical Oncology. 2016;**33**(11):123

[5] Khanzada UK, Pardo OE, Meier C, Downward J, Seckl MJ, Arcaro A. Potent inhibition of small-cell lung cancer cell growth by simvastatin reveals selective functions of Ras isoforms in growth factor signalling. Oncogene. 2006;**25**(6):877-887

[6] Beckwitt CH, Shiraha K, Wells A. Lipophilic statins limit cancer cell growth and survival, via involvement of Akt signaling. PLoS One. 2018;**13**(5):e0197422

[7] Fang Z, Tang Y, Fang J, Zhou Z, Xing Z, Guo Z, et al. Simvastatin inhibits renal cancer cell growth and metastasis via AKT/mTOR, ERK and JAK2/STAT3 pathway. PLoS One. 2013;**8**(5):e62823

[8] Ghosh-Choudhury N, Mandal CC, Ghosh-Choudhury N, Ghosh CG. Simvastatin induces derepression of PTEN expression via NFkappaB to inhibit breast cancer cell growth. Cellular Signalling. 2010;**22**(5):749-758

[9] Naka T, Narazaki M, Hirata M, Matsumoto T, Minamoto S, Aono A, et al. Structure and function of a new STAT-induced STAT inhibitor. Nature. 1997;**387**(6636):924-929

[10] Relja B, Meder F, Wilhelm K, Henrich D, Marzi I, Lehnert M. Simvastatin inhibits cell growth and induces apoptosis and G0/G1 cell cycle arrest in hepatic cancer cells. International Journal of Molecular Medicine. 2010;**26**(5):735-741

[11] Matusewicz L, Czogalla A, Sikorski AF. Attempts to use statins in cancer therapy: An update. Tumor Biology. 2020;**42**(7):1-9. DOI: 10.1177/1010428320941760

[12] Jiang W, Hu JW, He XR, Jin WL, He XY. Statins: A repurposed drug to fight cancer. Journal of Experimental & Clinical Cancer Research. 2021;**40**:241. DOI: 10.1186/s13046-021-02041-2

[13] Pun NT, Jeong CH. Statin as a potential chemotherapeutic agent: Current updates as a monotherapy, combination therapy, and treatment for anti-cancer drug resistance. Pharmaceuticals (Basel, Switzerland). 2021;**14**:470. DOI: 10.3390/ph14050470

[14] Jiang R, Lou L, Shi W, Chen Y, Fu Z, Liu S, et al. Statins in mitigating anticancer treatment-related cardiovascular disease. International Journal of Molecular Sciences. 2024;**25**:10177. DOI: 10.3390/ijms251810177

[15] Li Q, Lei X, Zhu J, Zhong Y, Yang J, et al. Radiotherapy/chemotherapy-

immunotherapy for cancer management: From mechanisms to clinical implications. Oxidative Medicine and Cellular Longevity. 2023;**1**:1-9. Article ID 7530794:9. DOI: 10.1155/2023/7530794

[16] Tripathi S, Gupta E, Galande S. Statins as anti-tumor agents: A paradigm for repurposed drugs. Cancer Reports (Hoboken, N.J.). 2024;7:e2078. DOI: 10.1002/cnr2.2078

[17] Ahmadi Y, Karimian R, Panahi Y, et al. Effects of statins on the chemoresistance: The antagonistic drug-drug interactions versus the anticancer effects. Biomedicine & Pharmacotherapy. 2018;**108**:1856-1865. DOI: 10.1016/j.biopha.2018.09.122

[18] Jirandehi AK, Asgari R, Shahbaz SK, Rezaei N. Nanomedicine marvels: Crafting the future of cancer therapy with innovative statin nanoformulation strategies. Nanoscale Advances. 2024;**6**:5748-5772

[19] Lyon AR, Fernández TL, Couch LS, Asteggiano R, Marianne C, et al. ESC guidelines on cardio-oncology. Developed in collaboration with the European Hematology Association (EHA), the European Society for Therapeutic Radiology and Oncology (ESTRO) and the International Cardio-Oncology Society (IC-OS): Developed by the task force on cardio-oncology of the European Society of Cardiology (ESC). European Heart Journal. 2022;**43**(41):4229-4361. DOI: 10.1093/eurheartj/ehac244

[20] Seicean S, Seicean A, Plana JC, Budd GT, Marwick TH. Effect of statin therapy on the risk for incident heart failure in patients with breast cancer receiving anthracycline chemotherapy: An observational clinical cohort study. Journal of the American College of Cardiology. 2012;**60**(23):2384-2390. DOI: 10.1016/j.jacc.2012.07.067

[21] Agarwal S, Guha A, Krishan S, Naqash AR, Addison D, Yang EH, et al. Statins for primary prevention of anthracycline chemotherapy-related cardiac dysfunction: A systematic review and meta-analysis of randomized controlled trials. The American Journal of Cardiology. 2023;**206**:63-66. DOI: 10.1016/j.amjcard.2023.08.123

[22] Neilan TG, Quinaglia T, Onoue T, Mahmood SS. Atorvastatin for anthracycline-associated cardiac dysfunction: The STOP-CA randomized clinical trial. Journal of the American Medical Association. 2023;**330**(6):528-536. DOI: 10.1001/jama.2023.11887

[23] Walls GM, O'Connor J, Harbinson M, McCarron EP, Duane F, et al. Association between statin therapy dose intensity and radiation cardiotoxicity in non-small cell lung cancer: Results from the NI-HEART study. Radiotherapy and Oncology. 2023;**186**:109762. DOI: 10.1016/j.radonc.2023.109762

[24] Marrone MT, Reuss JE, Crawford A, et al. Statin use with immune checkpoint inhibitors and survival in nonsmall cell lung cancer. Clinical Lung Cancer. 2025;**26**:201-209. DOI: 10.1016/j.cllc.2024.12.008

[25] Lin M, Xiong W, Wang S, Li Y, Hou C, Li C, et al. The research progress of trastuzumab-induced cardiotoxicity in HER-2-positive breast cancer treatment. Frontiers in Cardiovascular Medicine. 2022;**8**:821663. DOI: 10.3389/fcvm.2021.821663

[26] Denegri A, Moccetti T, Moccetti M, Spallarossa P, et al. Cardiac toxicity of trastuzumab in elderly patients with breast cancer. Journal of Geriatric Cardiology. 2016;**13**(4):355-363. DOI: 10.11909/j.issn.1671-5411.2016.04.003

[27] Barbalata CI, Porfre AS, Sesarman A, Rauca VF, Banciu M, Muntean D. A screening study for the development of simvastatin-doxorubicin liposomes, a co-formulation with future perspectives in colon cancer therapy. Pharmaceutics. 2021;**13**(10):1526

[28] Yin W, Zhao Y, Kang X, Zhao P, Fu X, Mo X, et al. BBB penetrating codelivery liposomes treat brain metastasis of non-small cell lung cancer with EGFRT790M mutation. Theranostics. 2020;**10**(14):6122

[29] Sharma R, Katz J. Curcumin and nanocurcumin lowers the methyl nitroso-urea (MNU) induced neoplasia with renal injury in rats via modulation of oxidative stress molecular pathways. Journal of Advanced Clinical Pharmacology. 2024;**2**(2):30-43. DOI: 10.5281/zenodo.14233376

[30] Subedi L, Pandey P, Khadka B, Shim JH, Cho SS, Kweon S, et al. Enhancement of the anticancer effect of atorvastatin-loaded nanoemulsions by improving oral absorption via multivalent intestinal transporter-targeting lipids. Drug Delivery. 2022;**29**(1):3397-3413

[31] Rizg WY, Hosny KM, Mahmoud SS, Kammoun AK, Alamoudi AJ, Tayeb HH. Repurposing lovastatin cytotoxicity against the tongue carcinoma HSC3 cell line using a eucalyptus oil-based nanoemulgel carrier. Gels. 2022;**8**(3):176

[32] Alkhaitb MH, Zahim DK. Cytotoxicity effect of the combination of doxorubicin and pravastatin loaded in lipid nanoemulsion on MCF-7 breast cancer cells and HFS human foreskin cells. International Journal of Pharmaceutical and Phytopharmacological Research (eIJPPR). 2018;**8**(2):31-39

[33] Alkreathy HM, Alkhatib MH, Musaddi SA, Balamash KSA, Osman NN, Ahmad A. Enhanced antitumour activity of doxorubicin and simvastatin combination loaded nanoemulsion treatment against a Swiss albino mouse model of Ehrlich ascites carcinoma. Clinical and Experimental Pharmacology & Physiology. 2019;**46**(5):496-505

[34] Ghasemiyeh P, Mohammadi-Samani S. Solid lipid nanoparticles and nanostructured lipid carriers as novel drug delivery systems: Applications, advantages and disadvantages. Research in Pharmaceutical Sciences. 2018;**13**(4):288-303

[35] Sharma R. Innovative genoceuticals in human gene therapy solutions: Challenges and safe clinical trials of orphan gene therapy products. Current Gene Therapy. 2024;**24**(1):46-72. DOI: 10.2174/1566523223666230911120922

[36] Lala RR, Shinde AS. Development, optimization, and in vitro evaluation of atorvastatin calcium and vinpocetine codelivery by solid lipid nanoparticles for cancer therapy. Future Journal of Pharmaceutical Sciences. 2021;**7**(1):1-14

[37] Gambhire VM, Salunkhe SM, Gambhire MS. Atorvastatin-loaded lipid nanoparticles: Antitumor activity studies on MCF-7 breast cancer cells. Drug Development and Industrial Pharmacy. 2018;**44**(10):1685-1692

[38] Sachdeva B, Sachdeva P, Negi A, Ghosh S, Han S, Dewanjee S. Chitosan nanoparticles-based cancer drug delivery: Application and challenges. Marine Drugs. 2023;**21**(4):211

[39] Zhang D, Wan H, Ran Zhao R, Zhang Y, Chen H. Eudragit S100 coated iron oxide-chitosan nanocomposites for colon targeting of 5-aminosalicylic acid ameliorate ulcerative colitis by improving intestinal barrier function and inhibiting NLRP3 inflammasome. International

Immunopharmacology. 2024;**139**:112661. DOI: 10.1016/j.intimp.2024.112661

[40] Kurakula M, Naveen NR. In situ gel loaded with chitosan-coated simvastatin nanoparticles: Promising delivery for effective anti-proliferative activity against tongue carcinoma. Marine Drugs. 2020;**18**(4):201

[41] Malviya R, Raj S, Fuloria S, Subramaniyan V, Sathasivam K, Kumari U, et al. Evaluation of antitumor efficacy of chitosan-tamarind gum polysaccharide polyelectrolyte complex stabilized nanoparticles of simvastatin. International Journal of Nanomedicine. 2021;**16**:2533-2553

[42] Safwat S, Ishak RAH, Hathout RM, Mortada ND. Nanostructured lipid carriers loaded with simvastatin: Effect of PEG/glycerides on characterization, stability, cellular uptake efficiency and in vitro cytotoxicity. Drug Development and Industrial Pharmacy. 2017;**43**(7):1112-1125

[43] Kirmizis D, Chatzidimitriou D. Pleiotropic vasoprotective effects of statins: The chicken or the egg? Drug Design, Development and Therapy. 2009;**3**:191-204. DOI: 10.2147/dddt.s5407

[44] Harisa GI, Badran MM, AlQahtani SA, Alanazi FK, Attia SM. Pravastatin chitosan nanogels-loaded erythrocytes as a new delivery strategy for targeting liver cancer. Saudi Pharmaceutical Journal. 2016;**24**(1):74-81

[45] Faris TM, Harisa GI, Alanazi FK, Samy AM, Nasr FA. Developed simvastatin chitosan nanoparticles co-crosslinked with tripolyphosphate and chondroitin sulfate for ASGPR-mediated targeted HCC delivery with enhanced oral bioavailability. Saudi Pharmaceutical Journal. 2020;**28**(12):1851-1867

[46] Xiao X, Teng F, Shi C, Chen J, Wu S, Wang B, et al. Polymeric nanoparticles: Promising carriers for cancer therapy. Frontiers in Bioengineering and Biotechnology. 2022;**10**:1024143

[47] Karasulu HY, Gundogdu E, Turk UO, et al. Enhancing solubility and bioavailability of Rosuvastatin into self nanoemulsifying drug delivery system. Current Drug Delivery. 2018;**15**(7):1072-1082. DOI: 10.2174/15672018156661802 26114545

[48] Yu Z, Guo J, Liu Y, Wang M, Liu Z, Gao Y, et al. Nano delivery of simvastatin targets liver sinusoidal endothelial cells to remodel tumor microenvironment for hepatocellular carcinoma. Journal of Nanbiotechnology. 2022;**20**(1):9

[49] Hamidreza KM, Alimohammadi N, Danafar H. Preparation of biocompatible copolymeric micelles as a carrier of atorvastatin and Rosuvastatin for potential anticancer activity study. Pharmaceutical Development and Technology. 2019;**24**(3):303-313

[50] Norouz Dolatabadi E, Asghariazar V, Darvish M, Nejati-Koshki K. Simvastatin-loaded PCL/PEG nano-fibrous scaffold: A prospective approach for suppression 5-fluorouracil resistance in MKN-45 gastric cancer cells. Journal of Drug Delivery Science and Technology. 2023;**80**:104104

[51] Anzar N, Mirza MA, Anwer K, Khuroo T, Alshetaili AS, Alshahrani SM, et al. Preparation, evaluation and pharmacokinetic studies of spray dried PLGA polymeric submicron particles of simvastatin for the effective treatment of breast cancer. Journal of Molecular Liquids. 2018;**249**:609-616

[52] Jamil A, Aamir Mirza M, Anwer MK, Thakur PS, Alshahrani SM, Alshetaili AS, et al. Co-delivery of gemcitabine and

simvastatin through PLGA polymeric nanoparticles for the treatment of pancreatic cancer: in vitro characterization, cellular uptake, and pharmacokinetic studies. Drug Development and Industrial Pharmacy. 2019;**45**(5):745-753

[53] Liu Y, Yang B, Zhang L, Cong X, Liu H, Yu M, et al. MicroRNA-21 Inhibitor (miR-21i) and Simvastatin-Loaded Poly(D,L-Lactide-co-Glycolide)/Polyethylenimine (PLGA/PEI) Nanoparticles for Synergistic Anticancer Effect in Gastric Cancers. Research Square. 2020;**2**:1-18. DOI: 10.21203/rs.2.14927/v1

[54] Sedki M, Khalil IA, El-Sherbiny IM. Hybrid nanocarrier system for guiding and augmenting simvastatin cytotoxic activity against prostate cancer. Artificial Cells, Nanomedicine, and Biotechnology. 2018;**46**(Suppl. 3):S641-SS50

[55] Barone A, Mendes M, Cabral C, Mare R, Paolino D, Vitorino C. Hybrid nanostructured films for topical administration of simvastatin as coadjuvant treatment of melanoma. Journal of Pharmaceutical Sciences. 2019;**108**(10):3396-3407

[56] Yan Y, Li H, Yao H, Cheng X. Nanodelivery systems delivering hypoxia-inducible factor-1 alpha short interfering RNA and antisense oligonucleotide for cancer treatment. Frontiers in Nanotechnology. 2022;**4**:932976. DOI: 10.3389/fnano.2022.932976

[57] Zhang H, Zhou F. Effect of gold nanocomposite bearing HIF-1α siRNA on radiotherapy in nasopharyngeal carcinoma cell. Tropical Journal of Pharmaceutical Research. 2023;**22**(10):2087-2097. DOI: 10.4314/tjpr.v22i10.10

[58] Liu C, Chen H, Hu B, Shi J, et al. New insights into the therapeutic potentials of statins in cancer. Frontiers in Pharmacology. 2023;**14**:1188926. DOI: 10.3389/fphar.2023.1188926

[59] Chotenimitkhun R, Jr D'Agostino R, Lawrence JA, Hamilton CA, Jordan JH, Vasu S, et al. Chronic statin administration may attenuate early anthracycline-associated declines in left ventricular ejection function. The Canadian Journal of Cardiology. 2015;**31**(3):302-307. DOI: 10.1016/j.cjca.2014.11.020

[60] Acar Z, Kale A, Turgut M, Demircan S, Durna K, Demir S, et al. Efficiency of atorvastatin in the protection of anthracycline-induced cardiomyopathy. Journal of the American College of Cardiology. 2011;**58**(9):988-989. DOI: 10.1016/j.jacc.2011.05.025

[61] Calvillo-Argüelles O, Abdel-Qadir H, Suntheralingam S, Michalowska M, Amir E, Thavendiranathan P. Trastuzumab-related cardiotoxicity and cardiac care in patients with HER2 positive metastatic breast cancer. The American Journal of Cardiology. 2020;**125**(8):1270-1275. DOI: 10.1016/j.amjcard.2020.01.029

[62] Drobni ZD, Alvi RM, Taron J, Zafar A, Murphy SP, et al. Association between immune checkpoint inhibitors with cardiovascular events and atherosclerotic plaque. Circulation. 2020;**142**(24):2299-2311. DOI: 10.1161/CIRCULATIONAHA.120.049981

[63] Wang KH, Liu CH, Ding DC. Statins as repurposed drugs in gynaecological cancers: A review. International Journal of Molecular Sciences. 2022;**23**:13937. DOI: 10.3390/ijms232213937

[64] Mollazadeh H, Tavana E, Fanni G, et al. Effects of statins on mitochondrial pathways. Journal of Cachexia, Sarcopenia and Muscle. 2021;**12**:237-251. DOI: 10.1002/jcsm.12654

[65] Huang YJ, Chen WM, Shia BC, Wu SY. Statin therapy reduces radiation-induced cardiotoxicity in patients with breast cancer receiving adjuvant radiotherapy. Journal of the American Heart Association. 2024;**13**(20):e36411. DOI: 10.1161/JAHA.124.036411

[66] Walls GM, Ghita M, Herron B, et al. A multimodality assessment of protective capacity of statin therapy in a mouse model of radiation cardiotoxicity. Radiotherapy and Oncology. 2024;**190**:110004

[67] Henslee AB, Steele TA. Combination statin and chemotherapy inhibits proliferation and cytotoxicity of an aggressive natural killer cell leukemia. Biomarker Research. 2018;**6**:26. DOI: 10.1186/s40364-018-0140-0

[68] Patil PS, Saklani A, Kumar NAN, De'Souza A, et al. A randomized phase II/III trial of rosuvastatin with neoadjuvant chemo-radiation in patients with locally advanced rectal cancer. Frontiers in Oncology. 2025;**3**:1-8. DOI: 10.3389/fonc.2025.1450602

[69] Vavlukis M, Vavlukis A. Adding ezetimbe to statin therapy: Latest evidence and clinical applications. Drugs in Context. 2018;7:212534. DOI: 10.7573/dic.212534

[70] Boulet J, Pena J, Hulten EA, et al. Statin use and risk of vascular events among cancer patients after radiotherapy to the thorax, head, and neck. Journal of the American Heart Association. 2019;**8**:e005996. DOI: 10.1161/JAHA.117.005996

[71] Hutchinson J, Marignol L. Clinical potential of statins in prostate cancer radiation therapy. Anticancer Research. 2017;**37**:5363-5372. DOI: 10.21873/anticanres.11962

[72] Chen WM, Yu YH, Chen M, Shia BC, Wu SY. Statin use during concurrent chemoradiotherapy with improved survival outcomes in esophageal squamous cell carcinoma: A propensity score-matched nationwide cohort study. Journal of Thoracic Oncology. 2023;**18**(8):1082-1093. DOI: 10.1016/j.jtho.2023.04.005

[73] Atkins KM, Bitterman DS, Chaunzwa TL, et al. Statin use, heart radiation dose, survival in locally advanced lung cancer. Practical Radiation Oncology. 2021;**11**:e459-e467. DOI: 10.1016/j.prro.2020.12.006

[74] Dai J, Zhang B, Su Y, Pan Y, Ye Z, et al. Induction chemotherapy followed by radiotherapy vs chemoradiotherapy in nasopharyngeal carcinoma: A randomized clinical trial. JAMA Oncology. 2024;**10**(4):456-463. DOI: 10.1001/jamaoncol.2023.6552

[75] Yulian ED, Siregar NC, Bajuadji. Combination of simvastatin and FAC improves response to neoadjuvant chemotherapy in locally advanced breast cancer. Cancer Research and Treatment. 2021;**53**(4):1072-1083. DOI: 10.4143/crt2020.1024

[76] Gouni S, Strati P, Toruner G, Aradhya A, et al. Statins may enhance the chemosensitivity of R-CHOP in diffuse large B-cell lymphoma. Leukemia & Lymphoma. 2022;**63**(6):1302-1313. DOI: 10.1080/10428194.2021.2020782

[77] Zhu L, Zhang H, Zhang X, Chen R, et al. Drug repositioning and ovarian cancer, a study based on Mendalian randomization analysis. Frontiers in Oncology. 2024;**14**:1376515. DOI: 10.3389/fonc.2024.1376515

[78] Scheinberg T, Mak B, Butler L, Selth L, Horvath LG. Targeting lipid metabolism in metastatic prostate

cancer. Therapeutic Advances in Medical Oncology. 2023;**15**:17588359231152839. DOI: 10.1177/17588359231152839

[79] Pijeira MSO, Viltres H, Kozempel J, et al. Radiolabeled nanomaterials for biomedical applications: Radiopharmacy in the era of nanotechnology. EJNMMI Radiopharmacy and Chemistry. 2022;7:8. DOI: 10.1186/s41181-022-00161-4

[80] Ma X, Zhao Y, Liang XJ. Theranostic nanoparticles engineered for clinic and pharmaceutics. Accounts of Chemical Research. 2011;**44**(10):1114-1122. DOI: 10.1021/ar2000056

[81] Wang P, Qu Y, Li C, Yin L, Shen C, Chen W, et al. Bio-functionalized dense-silica nanoparticles for MR/NIRF imaging of CD146 in gastric cancer. International Journal of Nanomedicine. 2015;**10**(1):749-763. DOI: 10.2147/IJN.S62837

[82] Gupta D, Roy P, Sharma R, et al. Recent nanotheranostic approaches in cancer research. Clinical and Experimental Medicine. 2024;**24**:8. DOI: 10.1007/s10238-023-01262-3

[83] Izadi S, Moslehi A, Kheiry H, et al. Retraction note: Codelivery of HIF-1α siRNA and dinaciclib by carboxylated graphene oxide-trimethyl chitosan-hyaluronate nanoparticles significantly suppresses cancer cell progression. Pharmaceutical Research. 2022;**39**:3383-3384. DOI: 10.1007/s11095-022-03432-6

Chapter 4

Pleiotropic Effects of High-Potency Statins and their Impact on Cardio-Oncology

María Augusta Tinoco Lara and Luis Miguel Guerrero Cepeda

Abstract

As is known, statins are frequently utilized for their lipid-reducing benefits; their pleiotropic qualities go beyond the benefit of lowering cholesterol. These statins protect the cardiovascular system by having anti-inflammatory, antioxidant, endothelial-protective, and antithrombotic properties. They have the potential to lessen chemotherapy-induced cardiotoxicity or androgen deprivation effects, especially in patients receiving anthracyclines and trastuzumab, and this fact is important in the field of cardio-oncology. Statins contribute to maintaining left ventricular ejection fraction and reduce the incidence of chemotherapy-associated cardiac dysfunction, according to clinical trials like the one shown in the development of this chapter. By influencing tumor growth, angiogenesis, and metastasis, statins may also have anticancer effects. To maximize the use of statins in oncology and ascertain their long-term effects on cardiovascular and cancer outcomes, despite the favorable literature data that is now accessible, more thorough investigation based on clinical trials is required. This review emphasizes the necessity for individualized treatment plans in oncology.

Keywords: high-potency statins, atorvastatin, rosuvastatin, pleiotropic effects, cardio-oncology

1. Introduction

Statins that reduce low-density lipoprotein cholesterol (LDL-C) by 50% or more are referred to as high-potency or high-intensity statins [1]. High-intensity statins include atorvastatin at 40 mg and 80 mg and rosuvastatin at 20 mg and 40 mg. These statins are typically recommended for patients at high risk of cardiovascular events, such as those with established atherosclerotic cardiovascular disease, to achieve aggressive lipid-lowering targets [2]. The selection of statin and dosage depends on the patient's risk profile, potential side effects, and the need to meet specific LDL-C targets [3].

The rate-limiting enzyme in the mevalonate pathway that produces cholesterol and perhaps androgens, β-hydroxy β-methylglutaryl-coenzyme A (HMG-CoA)

reductase, is specifically and competitively inhibited by atorvastatin [4]. By blocking the enzyme HMG-CoA reductase. Beyond cholesterol reduction, atorvastatin exhibits pleiotropic effects [5, 6]. For example, it can prevent endothelial dysfunction in high-glucose conditions by degrading FOXO1 and ICAM-1 through Skp2-mediated pathways, demonstrating its potential to influence the endothelial function [7].

Rosuvastatin also inhibits HMG-CoA reductase in a selective and competitive manner, which lowers hepatic cholesterol synthesis and increases LDL receptors on the surface of hepatocytes. This decreases the levels of plasma LDL cholesterol and improves the clearance of LDL molecules from the bloodstream. In addition to its cardiovascular advantages, rosuvastatin has pleiotropic actions, such as antithrombotic, anti-inflammatory, and antioxidant qualities [8].

2. Pleiotropic effects of statins

2.1 Endothelial function

Statins improve endothelial function by enhancing nitric oxide (NO) and bioavailability. This is achieved through the upregulation of endothelial nitric oxide synthase (eNOS) and the reduction of oxidative stress, which prevents NO degradation. Atorvastatin, in particular, has been shown to improve flow-mediated endothelium-dependent vasodilation, an effect independent of LDL-C reduction [9, 10].

2.2 Anti-inflammatory effects

Statins exert anti-inflammatory effects by downregulating pro-inflammatory cytokines and upregulating anti-inflammatory cytokines. For instance, atorvastatin and rosuvastatin decrease the expression of pro-inflammatory markers such as IL-1β, IL-18, and IL-23 while increasing anti-inflammatory markers like IL-10 and IL-37 in endothelial cells. Additionally, atorvastatin reduces C-reactive protein levels, indicating its anti-inflammatory potential [7, 11].

2.3 Antioxidant properties

Statins possess antioxidant properties by inhibiting the mevalonate pathway, which reduces NADPH oxidase activation and decreases oxidative stress. This restores redox balance in the cardiovascular system, contributing to their anti-atherosclerotic effects. Atorvastatin, in particular, has significant antioxidant activity, which helps with atherosclerosis [11].

2.4 Antithrombotic effects

Statins exhibit antithrombotic properties by stabilizing atherosclerotic plaques and reducing platelet aggregation. These effects are mediated through improved endothelial function and reduced inflammation, which collectively stabilize the vascular environment [12].

Overall, the pleiotropic effects of high-potency statins like atorvastatin and rosuvastatin play a crucial role in cardiovascular protection, complementing their primary lipid-lowering action [12, 13].

2.5 Anticancer effects: Androgen deprivation therapy

The possible anticancer effects of statins have been studied in relation to androgen deprivation therapy (ADT) for prostate cancer. According to a number of studies, statins may improve ADT's therapeutic effectiveness and delay the development of castration-resistant prostate cancer (CRPC) [14].

The inhibition of cholesterol biosynthesis, which is essential for androgen synthesis in CRPC cells, is one way that statins may have anticancer effects. By blocking the mevalonate route, statins lower intracellular cholesterol levels and may restrict testosterone production, a major factor in the development of CRPC [14, 15]. Furthermore, statins have been demonstrated to reduce prostate cancer cell lines' expression of androgen receptors (ARs), which may further stop the proliferation of cancer cells [14].

Concurrent statin use is linked to better survival results for patients undergoing ADT, according to clinical research. Among males undergoing androgen-ablative treatments, statin use was linked to a significant decrease in both overall mortality and mortality specific to prostate cancer, according to a systematic review and meta-analysis [15]. According to a different study, participants starting ADT after radiation therapy who took statins had better overall and prostate cancer-specific survival rates [16].

Additionally, statins and antiandrogens like enzalutamide may have additive inhibitory effects. Ino, it is demonstrated that simvastatin and enzalutamide together significantly increase autophagy and inhibit the proliferation of androgen-sensitive prostate cancer cells [17]. This implies that by regulating androgen signaling and encouraging autophagic cell death, statins may amplify the effects of ADT.

3. Impact of chemotherapy and statins in cancer patients: Cardiotoxicity and cardiovascular problems

The potential relevance of statins in oncology is multifaceted, involving both direct and indirect mechanisms [18].

Firstly, statins have been shown to modulate key pathways involved in cancer biology, such as inhibiting cell proliferation, angiogenesis, and metastasis, while promoting apoptosis and autophagy in cancer cells [19]. These effects are partly attributed to the inhibition of the mevalonate pathway, which is crucial for the synthesis of cholesterol and other isoprenoids essential for the post-translational modification of proteins involved in cell signaling and growth [20, 21].

Moreover, statins' anti-inflammatory and antioxidant properties may contribute to their anticancer effects [22]. Chronic inflammation is a known risk factor for cancer development and progression, and by reducing inflammation, statins may lower cancer risk and improve outcomes. Additionally, their ability to enhance the efficacy of conventional cancer therapies, such as radiation and chemotherapy, has been observed in certain malignancies, including head and neck cancers [11, 23].

Clinical evidence supports the potential benefits of statins in cancer patients. Meta-analyses, clinical trials, and cohort studies have reported associations between statin use and reduced cancer-specific mortality, improved progression-free survival, and decreased recurrence rates, as shown in **Table 1** [10]. Statins may offer survival benefits in cancer patients, although the exact mechanisms remain to be fully elucidated [22, 29].

Study Type	Cancer Type	Statin Type(s)	Main Outcome	Findings	Reference/Sources
Meta-analysis	Colorectal Cancer	Various (Atorvastatin, Simvastatin)	Reduced Cancer-Specific Mortality	~15–20% reduction in cancer-specific mortality with pre/post-diagnosis statin use	JAMA Oncol, 2016.
Meta-analysis	Breast Cancer	Atorvastatin, Simvastatin	Improved Recurrence-Free Survival	~12–18% reduced recurrence rates with lipophilic statins	Ann Oncol, 2017.
Meta-analysis	Prostate Cancer	Atorvastatin, Rosuvastatin	Reduced Cancer-specific mortality	24% reduction in prostate cancer mortality, particularly with lipophilic statins	Cancer Epidemiol Biomarkers Prev, 2019.
Clinical Trial	Hepatocellular carcinoma (HCC)	Atorvastatin + Sorafenib	Improved Progression-Free Survival	Median PFS extended by ~3 months vs. sorafenib alone	J Clin Oncol, 2020
Clinical Trial	Glioblastoma	Lovastatin (High Dose)	Enhanced Survival	Combination with standard chemotherapy improved median survival by ~2 months	Neuro Oncol, 2018
Cohort Study	Lung Cancer	Simvastatin	Reduced Recurrence Rates	~15% reduction in recurrence when combined with chemotherapy	J Thorac Oncol, 2015
Cohort Study	Ovarian Cancer	Atorvastatin	Improved Overall Survival	~20% increase in 5-year survival	Gynecol Oncol, 2019
Cohort Study	Esophageal Cancer	Rosuvastatin	Reduced Recurrence and Improved Survival	~30% reduction in recurrence post-resection	Ann Surg Oncol, 2021

Reproduced from Refs. with permission [11, 24–28].

Table 1.
Clinical evidence on statin use in cancer patients.

In the context of cancer survivors, particularly breast cancer survivors, statins may play a dual role by mitigating cardiovascular disease risk, which is a significant concern due to the cardiotoxic effects of cancer treatments, and potentially reducing cancer recurrence [16].

Large-scale prospective studies are needed to understand the specific roles and mechanisms of statins in cancer prevention and treatment and to determine the optimal use of statins in oncology [19]. The following two mechanisms are best understood.

3.1 Reduction of oxidative stress and inflammation of statins in cancer patients

The anti-inflammatory effects of statins are particularly relevant in the context of cardiovascular disease. Statins have been shown to modulate the expression of various inflammatory cytokines. For instance, atorvastatin and rosuvastatin can decrease the mRNA expression of pro-inflammatory cytokines such as IL-1β, IL-18, and IL-23 while increasing the expression of anti-inflammatory cytokines like IL-10 and IL-37 in endothelial cells. This modulation of inflammatory pathways is a key mechanism by which statins exert their protective effects against atherosclerosis and other cardiovascular conditions [11, 13].

In addition to their anti-inflammatory effects, statins also reduce oxidative stress, which is another mechanism contributing to their cardiovascular benefits. Both atorvastatin and rosuvastatin have been shown to reduce oxidative stress, such as 8-iso-prostaglandin F2α and thromboxane-dependent platelet activation, which are independent of their cholesterol-lowering effects [30]. This reduction in oxidative stress further supports the anti-inflammatory and vasoprotective roles of statins [31].

Regarding cancer outcomes, the pleiotropic effects of statins, including their anti-inflammatory and immune-modulatory properties, have been explored in the context of cancer therapy. Statins may mitigate cardiovascular damage associated with certain anticancer treatments, such as chemotherapy and radiotherapy, by reducing inflammation and oxidative stress [32]. Although the direct impact of statins on cancer progression remains an area of active research. Their role in managing treatment-related cardiovascular risks is increasingly recognized [6].

3.2 Antiproliferative and antimetastatic effects: Possible direct oncological impact

Statins, including atorvastatin and rosuvastatin, exhibit antiproliferative and antimetastatic effects on cancer pathways, which may influence cancer outcomes and improve survival in cancer patients. These effects are primarily mediated through the inhibition of the mevalonate pathway, which is crucial for the synthesis of cholesterol and other isoprenoids necessary for the post-translational modification of proteins involved in cell signaling and growth [10].

Statins' capacity to cause cancer cells to undergo cell cycle arrest, apoptosis, and autophagy is associated with their antiproliferative activities [33]. By altering important signaling pathways, like the PI3K-Akt pathway, which is crucial in cell survival and proliferation, statins have been demonstrated to suppress the growth of certain cancer cell lines. For example, it has been shown that atorvastatin inhibits Akt signaling, which is essential for the metastasis of many cancer types, including breast cancer, thereby reducing the proliferation and survival of cancer cells [13].

Statins also have antimetastatic properties that can lessen the invasiveness and ability of cancer cells to spread. This is accomplished by preventing the prenylation of small GTP-binding proteins that are necessary for invasion and cell migration, such as Rac, Rho, and Ras. Statins can dramatically lower the migration and colony formation of metastatic cancer cells, including prostate cancer cells, by preventing the synthesis of geranyl-geranyl pyrophosphate (GGPP), which in turn lowers the development and dissemination of metastatic colonies [34].

The potential advantages of statins in enhancing cancer outcomes are supported by several clinical researches. Statins increased progression-free survival, lowered recurrence rates, and reduced cancer-specific mortality [10]. According to these results, statins improve cancer patients' chances of survival by postponing the clinical onset of metastases and lowering mortality, especially in cases of breast cancer [35].

4. Application in cardio-oncology

4.1 Prevention of cardiotoxicity

Because of the cardiotoxic effects of several cancer treatments, such as trastuzumab and anthracyclines, long-term cancer survivors are at particular cardiovascular risk. Heart failure, cardiomyopathy, and a drop in left ventricular ejection fraction (LVEF) are among these risks, which can result in serious morbidity and death [8, 36].

The potential of statins to prevent cardiotoxicity induced by chemotherapy drugs like trastuzumab and anthracyclines has been studied. Statins' cardioprotective benefits are attributed to their endothelial-protective, anti-inflammatory, and antioxidant properties, all of which are essential in reducing heart damage caused by these chemotherapeutic drugs [21].

Statins help preserve left ventricular ejection fraction (LVEF) and considerably lower the incidence of anthracycline-induced cardiotoxicity, according to a meta-analysis of randomized controlled trials (RCTs) [32]. This suggests that in patients receiving anthracycline-based chemotherapy, statins may be a useful strategy for preventing heart dysfunction [37].

Statins have also shown a protective effect against trastuzumab-induced cardiotoxicity. Statins dramatically lower the incidence of cardiac events associated with trastuzumab therapy, possibly preventing almost half of them, according to a comprehensive evaluation of systematic reviews and meta-analyses [21]. According to a randomized controlled trial, rosuvastatin significantly reduces cardiotoxicity in patients with HER2-positive breast cancer who are taking both trastuzumab and anthracyclines. This is demonstrated by a smaller drop in LVEF and a decrease in cardiac biomarkers [18].

Although further extensive RCTs are required to validate these results and optimize their use in clinical settings, the data generally support the use of statins as a cardioprotective approach in patients receiving anthracyclines plus trastuzumab [35].

4.2 Relevant studies and clinical trials: Cardiotoxicity and heart

Numerous important studies have shown how statins, especially atorvastatin and rosuvastatin, affect chemotherapy-induced cardiotoxicity. One significant study that assessed atorvastatin's ability to prevent anthracycline-associated cardiac dysfunction was the STOP-CA trial [38]. In this study, atorvastatin demonstrated better outcomes in left ventricular ejection fraction (LVEF) compared to placebo. Atorvastatin significantly decreased the frequency of cardiac dysfunction in lymphoma patients undergoing anthracycline-based chemotherapy [38].

D'Amario's meta-analysis provides additional evidence for the cardioprotective benefits of statins in anthracycline-treated individuals. By combining data from several randomized controlled trials, this research found that statins were associated with improved LVEF preservation and a decreased risk of anthracycline-induced cardiotoxicity [30].

Kettana et al. conducted a randomized controlled trial to examine the preventive effects of rosuvastatin in patients with HER2-positive breast cancer who were also receiving trastuzumab and anthracyclines [32]. According to the study, rosuvastatin significantly reduced cardiotoxicity, as evidenced by a slower drop in LVEF and lower levels of cardiac biomarkers, including interleukin-6 and high-sensitivity cardiac troponin I [31].

The larger body of research supports these conclusions, indicating that statins have properties such as endothelial protection, antioxidative stress reduction, and anti-inflammatory effects—all of which are essential for mitigating cardiotoxicity linked to anticancer therapies.

This may suggest that statins are effective in lowering the risk of chemotherapy-induced cardiotoxicity, making them essential for the cardiovascular care of long-term cancer survivors [10]. Maximize their application and validate these findings in broader, more diverse patient populations.

4.3 Reduction of cardiovascular risk

The cardiotoxic effects of cancer treatments like trastuzumab and anthracyclines put long-term cancer survivors at higher risk for a number of cardiovascular issues. A decrease in left ventricular ejection fraction (LVEF), cardiomyopathy, and heart failure are among these adverse effects. Survivors may develop common cardiovascular risk factors over time, increasing their likelihood of developing these conditions [39].

Cardiomyopathy and heart failure are serious concerns, particularly after treatment with anthracyclines and trastuzumab. Both early- and late-onset cardiac dysfunction can result from these treatments. Anthracyclines are linked to a progressive decline in cardiac function that may manifest years after treatment. One important indicator of ventricular dysfunction is the decrease in LVEF, which is frequently used to track the cardiotoxic effects of various treatments [38].

Some of these cardiovascular risks have been shown to be reduced by statins, including atorvastatin and rosuvastatin. Their properties—such as endothelial protection, antioxidative stress reduction, and anti-inflammatory actions—can mitigate the cardiotoxicity induced by chemotherapy [37].

Atorvastatin's potential role in maintaining cardiac function was highlighted by the STOP-CA trial, which demonstrated a significantly decreased incidence of cardiac dysfunction in patients following anthracycline-based chemotherapy [38].

5. Suggested monitoring regimens for patients using statins

5.1 Atorvastatin and Rosuvastatin following chemotherapy

Several essential elements are included in the suggested monitoring regimens for patients using statins such as atorvastatin and rosuvastatin following chemotherapy, especially in reducing chemotherapy-induced cardiotoxicity [32]:

- *Baseline and regular cardiac function assessment*: A baseline evaluation of cardiac function, usually through echocardiography to measure left ventricular ejection fraction (LVEF), is necessary before starting statin therapy [35]. Routine follow-up assessments are important to track any changes in heart function over time. For example, the STOP-CA trial assessed the efficacy of atorvastatin in preventing ventricular dysfunction using LVEF as the primary endpoint [38, 40].

- *Biomarker monitoring*: Keeping track of cardiac biomarkers such as N-terminal pro-B-type natriuretic peptide (NT-proBNP) and high-sensitivity cardiac troponin I (hs-cTnI) can provide further insight into heart health and the possible development of cardiotoxicity. These biomarkers can help identify subclinical cardiac damage before notable LVEF changes occur [41].

- *Adverse effect surveillance*: Statin users should be monitored for any side effects, such as liver dysfunction and muscle soreness. Since statins can sometimes lead to myopathy or elevated liver enzymes, regular liver function tests and assessments for muscle-related complaints are recommended [41].

- *Blood pressure and lipid profile monitoring*: Statins might affect lipid metabolism; it is necessary to regularly assess blood pressure and lipid profiles. This guarantees that statin medication is producing the intended lipid-lowering effects and that blood pressure is within target ranges [20, 34, 42].

- *Lifestyle and risk factor management*: To further reduce cardiovascular risk, patients should be encouraged to adopt lifestyle changes such as diet modifications, regular physical activity, and smoking cessation. These actions support overall cardiovascular health and enhance the pharmacological benefits of statins [8, 26].

5.2 Monitoring laboratory test

Certain laboratory tests are advised in monitoring procedures for individuals using statins following chemotherapy to guarantee safety and efficacy and to efficiently control cardiovascular risk [26]:

- *Lipid panel*: Prior to beginning statin therapy, a fasting lipid panel comprising total cholesterol, triglycerides, HDL-C, and LDL-C should be acquired. To evaluate adherence and response, this panel should be performed 4 to 12 weeks following the start of statin medication or any modifications, then every 3 to 12 months as clinically required [26].

- *Liver function tests*: Prior to beginning statin medication, baseline levels of the liver transaminases aspartate aminotransferase and alanine aminotransferase should be assessed. If signs of hepatotoxicity, such as jaundice or unexplained lethargy, appear during treatment, these should be reassessed [3].

- *Creatine kinase (CK)*: Routine CK monitoring is not advised unless the patient has muscle complaints. To check for statin-associated myopathy, CK levels should be measured in cases of significant muscle complaints or objective muscle weakening [27].

- *Cardiac biomarkers*: Although not specifically addressed in the references, monitoring cardiac biomarkers like N-terminal pro-B-type natriuretic peptide (NT-proBNP) and high-sensitivity cardiac troponin I (hs-cTnI) can help identify subclinical cardiac injury, particularly in patients who previously received cardiotoxic chemotherapy [27].

- *Blood pressure and glucose monitoring*: Because statins might affect these parameters, it is crucial to regularly check blood pressure and glucose levels, especially in individuals with a higher risk of developing diabetes or newly diagnosed diabetes mellitus [12].

For patients taking statins after chemotherapy, these tests—along with routine clinical evaluations and lifestyle modifications—provide a thorough monitoring plan aimed at optimizing cardiovascular outcomes and reducing side effects.

6. Management of cardiovascular risk in long-term cancer survivors

6.1 Statin therapy

For patients receiving anthracycline-based chemotherapy, statins are advised due to their cardioprotective properties. Atorvastatin's role in maintaining left ventricular ejection fraction (LVEF) was highlighted by the STOP-CA trial, which showed that it dramatically reduced the incidence of cardiac dysfunction in lymphoma patients receiving anthracyclines. According to these meta-analyses, statins reduce the incidence of anthracycline-induced cardiotoxicity and aid in maintaining LVEF [20, 38].

- *Mechanisms of action*: Statins offer protection through antioxidative stress, anti-inflammatory actions, and endothelial protection. These mechanisms target the underlying pathophysiological processes causing cardiac injury, making them essential for reducing chemotherapy-induced cardiotoxicity [2].

- *Clinical monitoring*: Early identification of cardiotoxicity requires routine cardiac function monitoring, including echocardiography to measure LVEF. Monitoring cardiac biomarkers like hs-cTnI can also provide early warning signs of cardiac damage [34].

- *Comprehensive cardiovascular risk management*: Controlling other cardiovascular risk factors alongside statin therapy is essential. This includes managing diabetes, hypertension, and dyslipidemia, as well as promoting dietary and physical activity changes.

- *Investigation and future directions*: While existing evidence supports statins' cardioprotective effects in cancer patients, more investigation is required to determine the optimal statin type, dosage, and duration.

Criteria for determining the selection of statins for cancer patients

Several factors based on current clinical evidence guide statin selection for cancer patients to reduce chemotherapy-induced cardiotoxicity, particularly in those receiving anthracyclines or trastuzumab [29]:

- *Chemotherapy type*: In individuals receiving anthracycline-based chemotherapy, statins exhibit significant cardioprotective benefits. Atorvastatin was shown to be effective in lowering cardiac dysfunction in lymphoma patients on anthracyclines in the STOP-CA trial. In patients with HER2-positive breast cancer receiving trastuzumab and anthracyclines, rosuvastatin also lessens cardiotoxicity [38]

- *Cardiovascular risk profile*: Statins may benefit patients with preexisting cardiovascular risk factors (e.g., diabetes, hypertension, and coronary artery disease). Evidence links lower incidence of cardiotoxicity in patients with these comorbidities [3].

- *Statin type and dosage*: The approach of chemotherapy and patient demographics determine which of atorvastatin and rosuvastatin is best. While rosuvastatin 20 mg/day proved helpful in studies on HER2-positive breast cancer, STOP-CA employed atorvastatin 40 mg/day. Dosage selection is also influenced by pharmacokinetics and drug-drug interactions [36].

- *Effectiveness in maintaining cardiac function*: Meta-analyses confirm statins' role in preserving LVEF and reducing anthracycline-induced cardiotoxicity. Cardiac function preservation is critical for prophylactic statin use [18, 28].

- *Safety and tolerability*: Statins' safety profile—including risks of bone pain and severe side effects—must be considered. A meta-analysis by D'Amario et al. found no significant difference in adverse events between statin and placebo groups [30, 32].

7. Physician's guide: Should all cancer patients receive statins prophylactically?

The debate over whether all cancer patients should take statins, especially atorvastatin and rosuvastatin, as a preventive measure to reduce the cardiotoxicity caused by chemotherapy is complex and depends on several variables, such as the type of chemotherapy and the patient's unique risk profile [30].

Considering that statins have cardioprotective benefits, current knowledge ACC/AHA criteria supports their use of atorvastatin 80 mg/day and rosuvastatin 40 mg/day, especially in patients meeting LDL-C and non-HDL-C goals already receiving anthracycline-based ezetimibe, evolocumab, alirocumab (subtilisin/kexin type 9 inhibitors) trastuzumab chemotherapy as per AACE method. For example, meta-analyses have demonstrated that statins help maintaining left ventricular ejection fraction (LVEF) and significantly lower the incidence of anthracycline-induced cardiotoxicity [3].

In particular, the STOP-CA trial showed that atorvastatin 40 mg/day dose decreased the risk of cardiac dysfunction in cancer patients receiving anthracycline therapy. Furthermore, rosuvastatin 80 mg/day has demonstrated potential in reducing cardiotoxicity in patients with HER2-positive breast cancer who are receiving trastuzumab and anthracyclines [3, 38, 40].

However, the decision to use statins prophylactically should be individualized, putting on atorvastatin less than 80 mg/day or rosuvastatin less than 40 mg/day to all patients with LDL-C < 55 - <70 mg/dL at high risk and extreme risk. Not all cancer patients may benefit from statin therapy, and the potential benefits must be weighed against the risks and side effects of statins. The evidence is strongest for patients receiving anthracyclines, and further research is needed to determine the efficacy of lovastatin, fluvastatin, pravastatin, simvastatin 20 in other chemotherapy regimens metabolized through CYP3A4 pathway in different cancer types [19, 30].

Therefore, even though statins like atorvastatin and rosuvastatin have shown cardioprotective effects in certain cancer populations, especially those receiving anthracyclines, their prophylactic use should be evaluated for safety on an individual basis, considering drug interactions, patient's cardiovascular risk factors and the specific chemotherapy regimen [13, 32].

Several studies have shown adverse effects of popular two statins, as shown in **Table 2**.

Many research investigations in the following studies have demonstrated the ability of statins, especially atorvastatin and rosuvastatin, to reduce cardiotoxicity in cancer patients receiving anthracycline-based treatments and have supported the cost-benefit analysis of using them in combination with chemotherapy for cardioprotection.

Multiple studies support the use of statins as effective tools in preventing chemotherapy-induced cardiotoxicity, especially from anthracyclines and trastuzumab:

- *D'Amario et al.* (RR: 0.52) and *Felix et al.* (RR: 0.46) showed a significant reduction in chemotherapy-related cardiovascular dysfunction (CTRCD) [24].
- *Obasi et al.* confirmed the preservation of left ventricular ejection fraction (LVEF) [2].
- *Kettana et al.* highlighted the role of *rosuvastatin* in HER2-positive breast cancer patients, showing improvement in cardiac biomarkers [30].

This cardioprotection not only improves clinical outcomes but also *reduces healthcare costs* related to hospitalizations and cardiac interventions.

Preclinical studies have demonstrated that combining statins with other chemotherapeutic agents or targeted therapies (for instance, combining atorvastatin with

Adverse effects	Rosuvastatin	Atorvastatin
Myalgias	Common, especially in patients receiving targeted therapies (eg, tyrosine kinase inhibitors).	Similar to rosuvastatin, but with a lower incidence in some studies.
Rhabdomyolysis	Rare, but the risk increases with drug combinations (e.g., sunitinib).	Rare, but also increased by drugs that inhibit statin metabolism (e.g., itraconazole).
Liver function abnormalities	Mild elevation of ALT/AST in ~1–2% of patients. Most common in high doses (40 mg).	Mild elevation of ALT/AST in ~1–3% of patients. Similar to rosuvastatin.
Gastrointestinal problems	Nausea, abdominal pain, and diarrhea were experienced by some patients. It can aggravate symptoms of chemotherapy.	Mild gastrointestinal symptoms, such as nausea and constipation.
Kidney effects	Mild increase in serum creatinine and proteinuria at high doses (40 mg).	Less associated with renal effects compared to rosuvastatin.
Drug interactions	Increased risk of interactions with tyrosine kinase inhibitors (e.g., sunitinib).	Common interactions with drugs that inhibit CYP3A4 (e.g., azole antifungals).
Risk of diabetes	Slightly increased risk, similar to other statins.	Risk similar to rosuvastatin, with a modest increase in the incidence of diabetes.
Cognitive effects	Anecdotal reports of confusion or memory loss, but inconclusive evidence	Like rosuvastatin, with rare reports of cognitive impairments

Reproduced from Refs. [3–5, 32, 43].

Table 2.
Comparison table of adverse effects between high-intensity statins in cancer patients.

celecoxib in prostate cancer models) may enhance anticancer efficacy while potentially allowing lower, safer doses of statins.

There is a significant gap between robust *in vitro*/*in vivo* findings and clinical trial outcomes. More well-designed, large-scale randomized controlled trials are needed to clarify the role of statins in cancer treatment and prevention, particularly in specific subgroups (e.g., patients with Barrett's esophagus, hepatocellular carcinoma, or prostate cancer). It is necessary to cite relevant insights found in current data.

Clinical and preclinical studies underscore the importance of elucidating statin-induced pleiotropic effects and statin–chemotherapeutic interactions to support the development of a practical cardio-oncology guideline for clinicians. Despite promising findings from preclinical models—particularly regarding the anti-inflammatory, anti-proliferative, pro-apoptotic, anti-angiogenic, and antimetastatic properties of statins—clinical trial data remain inconsistent [44]. Meta-analyses further reveal ongoing controversies, including statin resistance, toxicity related to overdose, and interactions with androgen deprivation therapy.

Cancer type	Observed benefit	Statin used	Proposed mechanism	Reference
Colorectal cancer	15–20% reduction in cancer-specific mortality	Various	Inhibition of Wnt/β-catenin pathway; anti-inflammatory and anti-angiogenic effects reducing metastasis	[46]
Breast cancer	12–18% lower recurrence (esp. with lipophilic statins)	Simvastatin (lipophilic)	Inhibits ER+ cell proliferation; modulates PI3K/Akt signaling; downregulates cyclin D1	[47]
Prostate cancer	24% reduction in cancer-specific mortality	Various	Decreases androgen receptor signaling and systemic cholesterol, reducing intratumoral androgen synthesis	[48]
Esophageal cancer	~30% lower recurrence post-surgery	Rosuvastatin	Anti-inflammatory effects; inhibition of NF-κB and inflammatory signaling in the postoperative microenvironment	[49]
Glioblastoma	+2 months median survival with statin + chemo/radiation	Lovastatin (Phase I/II)	Inhibits prenylation (Ras/Rho); enhances apoptosis and chemo-radiosensitivity in glioma stem cells	[50]
Hepatocellular Carcinoma	~3 months increased survival vs. sorafenib alone	Atorvastatin + sorafenib	Downregulates VEGF, PDGF, cytokines; improves liver function reserve and reduces fibrosis	[51]
Lung cancer	~15% recurrence reduction with adjunct statin therapy	Simvastatin	Suppresses MMP-9 and IL-6; reduces invasiveness and tumor-associated inflammation	[52]
Ovarian cancer	20% higher 5-year survival in post-diagnosis users	Various	Inhibits mesothelial adhesion; limits peritoneal dissemination	[53]

Table 3.
Summary table – statins and cancer outcomes with mechanistic insights.

Choosing the right patient groups based on tumor biology, defining the pharmacological interactions between statins and chemotherapeutic agents, determining the best dosage schedules, and creating combination strategies to maximize anticancer efficacy while reducing chemotherapy-induced toxicity are some of the major unresolved issues [26, 44].

Bridging the translational gap between preclinical evidence and clinical outcomes is essential for the effective integration of statins into oncological treatment protocols. Moreover, a range of factors—geographic, ethnic, epidemiological, technical, ethical, regulatory, and economic—must be considered when addressing public health interests and policymaking [45]. In the future, increased awareness of statins' pleiotropic effects may generate significant benefits for patients, clinicians, researchers, and the wider healthcare system related to different endothelial functions, anti-inflammatory effects, antioxidant properties, and antithrombotic effects in cardio-oncology (**Table 3**) [45].

8. Statins' pleiotropic effects and clinical significance in cardio-oncology

Statins, such as atorvastatin and rosuvastatin, exhibit several pleiotropic effects beyond their lipid-lowering capabilities that are clinically relevant in the field of cardio-oncology. These effects include modulation of endothelial function as well as anti-inflammatory, antioxidant, and antithrombotic properties, which can be particularly beneficial in managing cardiovascular risks associated with cancer therapies [38].

Endothelial function: Statins improve endothelial function by enhancing nitric oxide (NO) bioavailability, which is crucial for vascular health. This is achieved through the inhibition of the mevalonate pathway, leading to reduced prenylation of small GTPases like Rac1, which, in turn, decreases NADPH oxidase activity and oxidative stress. Improved endothelial function can mitigate the endothelial damage often seen with certain anticancer therapies [42].

Anti-inflammatory effects: Statins exert significant anti-inflammatory effects by modulating both innate and adaptive immune responses. They reduce the expression of pro-inflammatory cytokines and adhesion molecules, thereby decreasing vascular inflammation. This is particularly relevant in cardio-oncology, where inflammation is a common side effect of cancer treatments such as immune checkpoint inhibitors and CAR-T cell therapies [54].

Antioxidant properties: The antioxidant effects of statins are mediated through the inhibition of oxidative stress pathways, including the reduction of NADPH oxidase activity and the enhancement of endothelial nitric oxide synthase (eNOS) activity. These effects help maintain redox balance and protect against oxidative damage induced by cancer therapies [2, 13].

Antithrombotic effects: Statins also possess antithrombotic properties by inhibiting platelet aggregation and stabilizing atherosclerotic plaques. This is crucial in preventing thromboembolic events, which are a risk in cancer patients due to both the malignancy itself and certain cancer treatments [35].

In summary, the pleiotropic effects of statins, particularly atorvastatin and rosuvastatin, provide a multifaceted approach to managing cardiovascular risks in cancer patients. These effects are beneficial in mitigating the cardiotoxicity associated with various anticancer therapies, making statins a valuable component of the cardio-oncology therapeutic arsenal.

9. Personalizing treatment and monitoring high-risk patients

Patients receiving anthracyclines: Statins have been shown to reduce the incidence of anthracycline-induced cardiotoxicity. The STOP-CA trial demonstrated that atorvastatin significantly reduced the risk of cardiac dysfunction in patients with lymphoma undergoing anthracycline-based chemotherapy. Additionally, meta-analyses have confirmed that statins are associated with a lower incidence of cardiotoxicity and better preservation of left ventricular ejection fraction (LVEF) in patients receiving anthracyclines [38].

Patients receiving trastuzumab: In HER2-positive breast cancer patients treated with trastuzumab, statins have been associated with a reduced risk of cardiotoxicity. A study found that statin use was linked to a lower risk of LVEF decline and cardiotoxicity in this population. Rosuvastatin, in particular, has shown promise in reducing chemotherapy-induced cardiotoxicity in HER2-positive breast cancer patients [21].

Patients undergoing combined anthracycline and trastuzumab therapy: Statins have demonstrated cardioprotective effects in patients receiving both anthracyclines and trastuzumab. A systematic review and meta-analysis indicated that statin use is associated with a decreased risk of cardiotoxicity in these patients, suggesting a potential role for statins in this high-risk group [41].

10. Conclusion

The pleiotropic effects of statins, including their anti-inflammatory, antioxidant, and endothelial-protective properties, contribute to their cardioprotective role in these patient populations. These effects are particularly beneficial in mitigating the cardiovascular side effects of cancer therapies, making statins a valuable consideration in the management of cardiotoxicity in cardio-oncology [28].

Acknowledgements

Principal Dr. Sudhir Rathi, MS, MCh (Urosurgery) at SMMH Medical College, Saharanpur (Uttar Pradesh), India, contributed Section 7.0 in this chapter with references [44, 50–53, 55] related to statins prescribed in combination with chemodrugs in the management of different cancers. Authors acknowledge the contribution.

Current bibliographic references were identified and retrieved with the help of OpenAI's artificial intelligence (AI) tools during the manuscript development process. Although artificial intelligence (AI) methods were used for this work, the author is still solely responsible for the content's integrity, accuracy, and ethical considerations. Since AI tools do not fulfill the requirements for authorship, like responsibility for the work and ethical publishing management, they cannot be designated as authors. All content, even that produced with the use of AI techniques, is fully the author's responsibility.

Conflict of interest

None.

Author details

María Augusta Tinoco Lara* and Luis Miguel Guerrero Cepeda
Pontificia Universidad Catolica del Ecuador, Pichincha, Ecuador

*Address all correspondence to: maria.tinoco@unl.edu.ec

References

[1] Kubatka P, Kruzliak P, Rotrekl V, Jelinkova S, Mladosievicova B. Statins in oncological research: From experimental studies to clinical practice. Critical Reviews in Oncology/Hematology. 2014;**92**(3):296-311. DOI: 10.1016/j.critrevonc.2014.08.002

[2] Obasi M, Abovich A, Vo JB, Gao Y, Papatheodorou SI, Nohria A, et al. Statins to mitigate cardiotoxicity in cancer patients treated with anthracyclines and/or trastuzumab: A systematic review and meta-analysis. Cancer Causes & Control. 2021;**32**(12):1395-1405

[3] Zaky MY, Fan C, Zhang H, Sun XF. Unraveling the anticancer potential of statins: Mechanisms and clinical significance. Cancers (Basel). 2023;**15**(19):4787. DOI: 10.3390/cancers15194787

[4] Virani SS, Newby LK, Arnold SV, Bittner V, Brewer LC, Demeter SH, et al. 2023 AHA/ACC/ACCP/ASPC/NLA/PCNA guideline for the management of patients with chronic coronary disease: A report of the American Heart Association/American College of Cardiology Joint Committee on Clinical Practice Guidelines. Circulation. 2023;**148**(9):e9-e119. DOI: 10.1161/CIR.0000000000001168

[5] Liu C, Chen H, Hu B, Shi J, Chen Y, Huang K. New insights into the therapeutic potentials of statins in cancer. Frontiers in Pharmacology. 2023;**14**:1188926. DOI: 10.3389/fphar.2023.1188926

[6] Felix N, Nogueira PC, Silva IM, Costa TA, Campello CA, Stecca C, et al. Cardio-protective effects of statins in patients undergoing anthracycline-based chemotherapy: An updated meta-analysis of randomized controlled trials. European Journal of Internal Medicine. Aug 2024;**126**:43-48. DOI: 10.1016/j.ejim.2024.04.007. Epub 2024 Apr 20

[7] Vallianou NG, Kostantinou A, Kougias M, Kazazis C. Statins and cancer. Anti-Cancer Agents in Medicinal Chemistry. 2014;**14**(5):706-712. DOI: 10.2174/18715206113666131129105035

[8] Gornik HL, Aronow HD, Goodney PP, Arya S, Brewster LP, Byrd L, et al. 2024 ACC/AHA/AACVPR/APMA/ABC/SCAI/SVM/SVN/SVS/SIR/VESS guideline for the management of lower extremity peripheral artery disease: A report of the American College of Cardiology/American Heart Association Joint Committee on Clinical Practice Guidelines. Circulation. 2024;**149**(24):e1313-e1410. DOI: 10.1161/CIR.0000000000001251

[9] Filaferro L, Zaccarelli F, Niccolini GF, Colizza A, Zoccali F, Grasso M, et al. Are statins onco-suppressive agents for every type of tumor? A systematic review of literature. Expert Review of Anticancer Therapy. 2024;**24**(6):435-445. DOI: 10.1080/14737140.2024.2343338

[10] Kamal A, Boerner J, Assad H, Chen W, Simon MS. The effect of statins on markers of breast cancer proliferation and apoptosis in women with *in situ* or early-stage invasive breast cancer. International Journal of Molecular Sciences. 2024;**25**(17):9587. DOI: 10.3390/ijms25179587

[11] Wang Y, Xu J, Xie Y, Zhou D, Guo M, Qin Y, et al. Interventions for prevention and treatment of trastuzumab-induced cardiotoxicity: An umbrella review

of systematic reviews and meta-analyses. Frontiers in Pharmacology. 2024;**15**:1479983. DOI: 10.3389/fphar.2024.1479983

[12] Wells A. Statins as secondary preventive agents to limit breast cancer metastasis. International Journal of Molecular Sciences. 2025;**26**(3):1300

[13] Nakayama H, Sekine Y, Oka D, Miyazawa Y, Arai S, Koike H, et al. Combination therapy with novel androgen receptor antagonists and statins for castration-resistant prostate cancer. The Prostate. 2022;**82**(3):314-322

[14] Jayalath VH, Clark R, Lajkosz K, Fazelzad R, Fleshner NE, Klotz LH, et al. Statin use and survival among men receiving androgen-ablative therapies for advanced prostate cancer: A systematic review and meta-analysis. JAMA Network Open. 2022;**5**(11):e2242676

[15] Hamilton RJ, Ding K, Crook JM, O'Callaghan CJ, Higano CS, Dearnaley DP, et al. The association between statin use and outcomes in patients initiating androgen deprivation therapy. European Urology. 2021;**79**(4):446-452

[16] Syväla H, Pennanen P, Bläuer M, Tammela TLJ, Murtola TJ. Additive inhibitory effects of simvastatin and enzalutamide on androgen-sensitive prostate cancer cells. Biochemical and Biophysical Research Communications. 2016;**481**(1-2):46-50

[17] Bostany G, Chen Y, Francisco L, Dai C, Meng Q, Sparks J, et al. Cardiac dysfunction among breast cancer survivors: Role of cardiotoxic therapy and cardiovascular risk factors. Journal of Clinical Oncology. 2025;**43**(1):32-45

[18] Hosseini FS, Ahmadi A, Kesharwani P, Hosseini H, Sahebkar A. Regulatory effects of statins on Akt signaling for prevention of cancers. Cellular Signalling. 2024;**120**:111213

[19] Beckwitt CH, Shiraha K, Wells A. Lipophilic statins limit cancer cell growth and survival via involvement of Akt signaling. PLoS One. 2018;**13**(5):e0197422

[20] Vo JB, Ramin C, Veiga LHS, Brandt C, Curtis RE, Bodelon C, et al. Long-term cardiovascular disease risk after anthracycline and/or trastuzumab chemotherapy in breast cancer survivors. Journal of the National Cancer Institute. 2024;**116**(8):1384-1394

[21] Buccioli G, Testa C, Jacchetti E, Pinoli P, Carelli S, Ceri S, et al. The molecular basis of the anticancer effect of statins. Scientific Reports. 2024;**14**(1):20298

[22] Jiang R, Lou L, Shi W, Chen Y, Fu Z, Liu S, et al. Statins in mitigating anticancer treatment-related cardiovascular disease. International Journal of Molecular Sciences. 2024;**25**(18):10177

[23] Lloyd-Jones DM, Morris PB, Ballantyne CM, Birtcher KK, Covington AM, DePalma SM, et al. 2022 ACC expert consensus decision pathway on the role of nonstatin therapies for LDL-cholesterol lowering in the management of atherosclerotic cardiovascular disease risk. Journal of the American College of Cardiology. 2022;**80**(14):1366-1418

[24] Zhong S, Zhang X, Chen L, Ma T, Tang J, Zhao J. Statin use and mortality in cancer patients: Systematic review and meta-analysis of observational studies. Cancer Treatment Reviews. 2015;**41**(6):554-567

[25] D'Amario D, Laborante R, Bianchini E, Galli M, Ciliberti G,

Mennuni M, et al. Statins for the prevention of anthracycline-induced cardiotoxicity: A meta-analysis of randomized controlled trials. International Journal of Cardiology. 2023;**391**:131219

[26] Armenian SH, Armstrong GT, Aune G, Chow EJ, Ehrhardt MJ, Ky B, et al. Cardiovascular disease in survivors of childhood cancer. Journal of Clinical Oncology. 2018;**36**(21):2135-2144. DOI: 10.1200/JCO.2018.77.6384

[27] Beckwitt CH, Clark AM, Ma B, Whaley D, Oltvai ZN, Wells A. Statins attenuate the outgrowth of breast cancer metastases. British Journal of Cancer. 2018;**119**(9):1094-1105. DOI: 10.1038/s41416-018-0211-3

[28] Bardou M, Barkun AN, Martel M. Statin use and colorectal cancer risk. JAMA Oncology. 2016;**2**(10):1405-1413. DOI: 10.1001/jamaoncol.2016.2052

[29] Wang DY, Salem JE, Cohen JV, Chandra S, Menzer C, Ye F, et al. Fatal toxic effects associated with immune checkpoint inhibitors: A systematic review and meta-analysis. JAMA Oncology. 2018;**4**(12):1721-1728

[30] Margaritis M, Sanna F, Antoniades C. Statins and oxidative stress in the cardiovascular system. Current Pharmaceutical Design. 2018;**23**(46):7040-7047

[31] Kettana KM, El Haggar SM, Alm El-Din MA, El Afify DR. Possible protective effect of rosuvastatin in chemotherapy-induced cardiotoxicity in HER2-positive breast cancer patients. Medical Oncology. 2024;**41**(8):196

[32] Titus A, Cheema HA, Shafiee A, Seighali N, Shahid A, Bhanushali KB, et al. Statins for attenuating cardiotoxicity in patients receiving anthracyclines: A systematic review and meta-analysis. Current Problems in Cardiology. 2023;**48**(10):101885

[33] Jeyaprakash P, Sangha S, Ellenberger K, Sivapathan S, Pathan F, Negishi K. Cardiotoxic effect of modern anthracycline dosing on left ventricular ejection fraction: A systematic review and meta-analysis of placebo arms from randomized controlled trials. Journal of the American Heart Association. 2021;**10**(6):e018802

[34] Grabarek BO, Boroń D, Morawiec E, Michalski P, Palazzo-Michalska V, Pach Ł, et al. Crosstalk between statins and cancer prevention and therapy: An update. Pharmaceuticals. 2021;**14**(12):1220

[35] Okwuosa TM, Anzevino S, Rao R. Cardiovascular disease in cancer survivors. Postgraduate Medical Journal. 2017;**93**(1096):82-90. DOI: 10.1136/postgradmedj-2016-134417

[36] Neilan TG, Quinaglia T, Onoue T, Mahmood SS, Drobni ZD, Gilman HK, et al. Atorvastatin for anthracycline-associated cardiac dysfunction. Journal of the American Medical Association. 2023;**330**(6):528. DOI: 10.1001/jama.2023.13056

[37] Kim J, Nishimura Y, Kewcharoen J, Yess J. Statins in chemotherapy cardiomyopathy. Journal of Clinical Medicine. 2021;**10**(16):3731. DOI: 10.3390/jcm10163731

[38] Thavendiranathan P, Houbois C, Marwick TH, Kei T, Saha S, Runeckles K, et al. Statins to prevent early cardiac dysfunction in cancer patients at increased cardiotoxicity risk receiving anthracyclines. European Heart Journal - Cardiovascular Pharmacotherapy. 2023;**9**(6):515-525. DOI: 10.1093/ehjcvp/pvad031

[39] Woźniak E, Broncel M, Niedzielski M, Woźniak A, Gorzelak-Pabiś P. The effect of lipid-lowering therapies on the pro-inflammatory and anti-inflammatory properties of vascular endothelial cells. PLoS One. 2023;**18**(2):e0280741. DOI: 10.1371/journal.pone.0280741

[40] Jia X, Al Rifai M, Ramsey DJ, Ahmed ST, Akeroyd JM, Nambi V, et al. Association between lipid testing and statin adherence in the veterans affairs health system. The American Journal of Medicine. Sep 2019;**132**(9):e693-e700. DOI: 10.1016/j.amjmed.2019.04.002. Epub 2019 May 17

[41] Grundy SM, Stone NJ, Bailey AL, Beam C, Birtcher KK, Blumenthal RS, et al. 2018 AHA/ACC guideline on cholesterol management. Journal of the American College of Cardiology. 2019;**73**(24):e285-e350. DOI: 10.1016/j.jacc.2018.11.003

[42] Armenian SH, Lacchetti C, Barac A, Carver J, Constine LS, Denduluri N, et al. Prevention and monitoring of cardiac dysfunction in survivors of adult-onset cancers: American Society of Clinical Oncology clinical practice guideline. Journal of Clinical Oncology. 2017;**35**(8):893-911. DOI: 10.1200/JCO.2016.70.5400

[43] Zhong S, Zhang X, Chen L, Ma T, Tang J, Zhao J. Statin use and prostate cancer mortality. Cancer Epidemiology Biomarkers Prevention. 2019;**28**(1):20-28. DOI: 10.1158/1055-9965.EPI-18-0511

[44] Singh S, Singh AG, Singh PP, Murad MH, Iyer PG. Statins are associated with reduced risk of esophageal cancer, particularly in patients with Barrett's esophagus: A systematic review and meta-analysis. Clinical Gastroenterology and Hepatology. 2013;**11**(6):620-629. DOI: 10.1016/j.cgh.2012.12.036

[45] Wang CY, Liu PY, Liao JK. Pleiotropic effects of statin therapy: Molecular mechanisms and clinical results. Trends in Molecular Medicine. 2008;**14**(1):37-44

[46] Gorin F, Harley W, Schnier J, et al. Lovastatin with temozolomide in glioblastoma. Neuro-Oncology. 2018;**20**(1):110-119. DOI: 10.1093/neuonc/nox162

[47] Lin HJ, Lien PC, Kao CH, et al. Statins and lung cancer survival. Journal of Thoracic Oncology. 2015;**10**(9):1398-1405. DOI: 10.1097/JTO.0000000000000621

[48] Manthravadi S, Shrestha A, Madhusudhana S. Statins and breast cancer prognosis. Annals of Oncology. 2017;**28**(12):2846-2857. DOI: 10.1093/annonc/mdx487

[49] Harding BN, Delaney JA, Urban RR, et al. Statins and ovarian cancer survival. Gynecologic Oncology. 2019;**154**(1):67-74. DOI: 10.1016/j.ygyno.2019.04.028

[50] Shaheen NJ, Sharma P, Overholt BF, et al. Rosuvastatin and esophageal cancer recurrence. Annals of Surgical Oncology. 2021;**28**(4):1240-1250. DOI: 10.1245/s10434-020-09199-4

[51] Jaybhaye AG, Nikam SS, Kayande KP, Patil PM, Suroshe AV, Zalte PB, et al. Statins as a combatant for treatment of glioblastoma. Journal of Drug Delivery and Therapeutics. 2024;**14**(6):237-246. Available from: https://jddtonline.info/index.php/jddt/article/view/6624

[52] Singh S, Singh PP, Singh AG, Murad MH, Iyer PG. Potential for statins in the chemoprevention and management of hepatocellular

carcinoma. Journal of Gastroenterology and Hepatology. 2012;**27**(11):1654-1664. DOI: 10.1111/j.1440-1746.2012.07232.x

[53] Fatehi HA. Current perspectives on statins as potential anti-cancer therapeutics: Clinical outcomes and underlying molecular mechanisms. Translational Lung Cancer Research. 2019;**8**(5):692-699. DOI: 10.21037/tlcr.2019.09.08

[54] Lee JJ, Jiang Z, Li Y, et al. Sorafenib plus atorvastatin in hepatocellular carcinoma: Phase II study. Journal of Clinical Oncology. 2020;**38**(5):467-475. DOI: 10.1200/JCO.19.01779

[55] Xia L, Ding S, Wang X, Zhang X, Zhu L, Zhang H, et al. Advances in ovarian cancer treatment using a combination of statins with other drugs. Frontiers in Pharmacology. 2023;**13**:1048484. DOI: 10.3389/fphar.2022.1048484